Davis's Physician's Drug Guide

Patricia R. Audet, Pharm.D.

Associate Professor of Clinical Pharmacy
Philadelphia College of Pharmacy and Science

F. A. DAVIS COMPANY • Philadelphia

Copyright © 1989 by F. A. Davis Company

All rights reserved. This book is protected by copyright. No part of it may be reproduced, stored in a retrieval system, or transmitted in any form or by any means, electronic, mechanical, photocopying, recording, or otherwise, without written permission from the publisher.

Printed in the United States of America

Last digit indicates print number: 10 9 8 7 6 5 4 3 2 1

NOTE: As new scientific information becomes available through basic and clinical research, recommended treatments and drug therapies undergo changes. The author(s) and publisher have done everything possible to make this book accurate, up-to-date, and in accord with accepted standards at the time of publication. However, the reader is advised always to check product information (package inserts) for changes and new information regarding dose and contraindications before administering any drug. Caution is especially urged when using new or infrequently ordered drugs.

Library of Congress Cataloging-in-Publication Data

Audet, Patricia R.
  Davis's physician's drug guide/Patricia R. Audet.
    p. cm. — (Essentials of medical education series)
  Includes bibliographies.
  Includes index.
  ISBN 0-8036-0451-3
  1. Drugs—Prescribing—Handbooks, manuals, etc. I. Title. II. Title: Physician's drug guide. III. Series.
  [DNLM: 1. Drugs—administration & dosage—handbooks. 2. Pharmacology—handbooks. 3. Prescriptions, Drug—handbooks. QV 39 A899d]
RM138.A83 1989
615'.1—dc19
DNLM/DLC
for Library of Congress   89-1627
                                                                        CIP

Authorization to photocopy items for internal or personal use, or the internal or personal use of specific clients, is granted by F. A. Davis Company for users registered with the Copyright Clearance Center (CCC) Transactional Reporting Service, provided that the fee of $.10 per copy is paid directly to CCC, 27 Congress St., Salem, MA 01970. For those organizations that have been granted a photocopy license by CCC, a separate system of payment has been arranged. The fee code for users of the Transactional Reporting Service is: 8036-0451/89 0 + $.10.

CONTENTS

The Importance of Prescribing Precisely
 by R. A. P. Burt, MB, ChB, FRCPE. **1**

Special Dosing Considerations **5**

Nomogram **11**

Schedules of Controlled Drugs **12**

Commonly Used Abbreviations **14**

**100 Most Frequently Prescribed
Hospital Drugs**
 by Pharmacologic Class **16**
 by Generic Name **19**

Alphabetical Listing of Generic Drugs . . .   **21–136**
 NOTE: The most common side
 effects/adverse reactions are printed in
 boldface type.

Index **137**

THE IMPORTANCE OF PRESCRIBING PRECISELY

R. A. P. BURT, MB, ChB, FRCPE

In 1892, *The Principles and Practice of Medicine*, written by Sir William Osler, Professor of Medicine at Johns Hopkins University, became the standard textbook of medicine. Yet only 10 percent of the entire book dealt with treatment. This was not willful therapeutic nihilism but forced practical necessity. Physicians of the day had very few effective drugs with which to treat their patients, and most of these were of herbal origin, the Poppy, Foxglove, Cinchona, and Willow. Most of the practice of Medicine consisted of diagnosis, giving the disease an eponymous identity, and disguising one's therapeutic impotence by an elaborately arcane prescription. Treatment consisted of prescribing elegantly concocted solutions, draughts, potions, tinctures, balms, and salves—almost all of them ineffective, but harmless. No wonder that Oliver Wendell Holmes—physician, lawyer, humorist, and Dean of Harvard Medical School—could write, "Throw out opium—throw out a few specifics which our art did not discover—throw out wine—and I firmly believe that if the whole materia medica, as now used, could be sunk to the bottom of the sea, it would be all the better for mankind—and all the worse for the fishes." How the physicians must have envied their surgical colleagues, for the advent of anesthesia and antisepsis heralded a period of unprecedented surgical achievement.

A century later much has changed, yet almost the whole medical curriculum remains concentrated on diagnosis. We live in the therapeutic revolution, but formal teaching of therapeutics has not kept pace, and the teaching of prescription writing is ignored in many medical schools. When I was a medical student, our professor of therapeutics often warned us of the potency of modern drugs.[3] He described them picturesquely and memorably as "the therapeutic thunderbolts of Jove" and encouraged us to treat them with respect.

Drugs produce their effects by disturbing the patient's internal milieu and, as Newton's third law—that's the one about actions producing equal and opposite reactions—predicts, the body reacts with different physiological responses. Professor Dunlop would explain the ubiquity of these effects by saying, "Show me a drug without side effects, and I'll show you a drug without any effect." Many problems of therapy, either lack of efficacy or adverse events, can be traced to inadequate prescription instructions, and you must be careful to avoid the simplistic sophism of post hoc, ergo propter hoc. Although it is true that we all will die sometime *after* our last meal, very few of us will die *because* of our last meal.

Prescribing a modern drug to treat a patient is equivalent to recommending a surgical procedure and deserves the same care. Most hospital physicians will write a prescription but leave to a nurse the actual administration of the drug to the patient. Because the prescriber usually is not present when the drug is given, clear instructions are paramount.

WHAT TO INCLUDE ON THE CHART ORDER OR PRESCRIPTION

The Date

Always include the date. It may be crucial to know when the drug is to be started, how long the drug has been taken, or if two drugs were given concomitantly.

R

This symbol (not Rx!) stands for recipe, meaning "take," and used to identify for the pharmacist those elements to be compounded in the mixture. Nowadays it identifies the drug to be supplied. Because many drug names, either generic or proprietary, may appear to be similar, I recommend that you print the DRUG NAME CLEARLY. Be sure to specify the dose or strength, especially if a solution or suspension is to be diluted for pediatric or elderly patients. The effects from the wrong dose may be as devastating as those from the wrong surgery and may even require surgical intervention to correct them.

Sig.

This is an abbreviation for "signa," meaning mark or write, and specifies the instructions to accompany the medication. Even if you have explained everything to the patient, these written instructions should be absolutely clear and unambiguous. Patients tend to be upset by illness, are often confused by, or unable to comprehend, the physician's explanation, and forget what they are told—especially if they are elderly. They may be taking several drugs, and a number of similar tablets can easily be mixed up in terms of dose and frequency of dosing.

The words, "Take as directed" are a prescription for disaster and should never appear. Use simple English, avoid jargon, and if the patient is taking several drugs, identify each one simply, for example, tablets for headache, capsules for blood pressure. Use correct grammar to avoid humiliations such as "Take the tablets as directed by the physician in water."

It is important to specify the frequency with which the drug should be taken. This becomes critical if it is necessary to take the drug with food to reduce the risk of gastric upset, or to avoid food because it impairs drug absorption, as with tetracyclines.

Signature

Always sign your prescription. Not only is this a legal requirement, it should foster caution because responsibility can be identified.

Scheduled Drugs

It is important to remember how often you need to rewrite prescriptions for scheduled drugs (see p. XX).

SOME INCOMPATIBILITIES

Although you may be meticulous in writing your prescription, there are still one or two traps to be avoided.

Physical Incompatibility

I recommend only one drug per prescription to prevent misunderstanding. However, if two drugs are prescribed concomitantly, consider whether or not they are physically compatible, for instance, in the same infusion solution, or will one cause precipitation of the other?

Pharmacological Incompatibility

Even if only one drug is prescribed, it is critical to ascertain what other drugs the patient may be taking. Considering only a few of the 100 drugs listed in this book, for example, cimetidine may reduce hepatic blood flow and inhibit the metabolism of propranolol. Phenobarbital will induce the enzymes that metabolize warfarin, leading to reduced anticoagulant activity. Quinidine may displace digoxin from myocardial stores, leading to digoxin toxicity. Surgery will delay postoperative gastric emptying, with delayed absorption of drugs given orally.

Verbal Incompatibility

Avoid jargon and abbreviations. If written hurriedly, "as" (auris sinister) can look like "os" (oculus sinister). With dosing frequency, the problem can get worse.[1] The Latin abbreviations "bid," "tid," and "qid" are commonly used, and if more specific timing is required a mixture of Latin and English is concocted, for example, "q 8 h" or "q 12 h." A dilemma arises with a prescription for a single dose. The Latin "unique" seems cumbersome and the abbreviation "u" is unfamiliar, so many physicians resort to "OD." Unfortunately, this particular abbreviation is used in several branches of medicine and means different things to different people.

A mixture of English and Latin offers opportunities for confusion between "one dose," "once daily," or "every day" (omni die). With patient-controlled analgesia, it might be reasonable to prescribe the drug "on demand." Ophthalmologists apply drugs topically, "one drop" at a time. Because application may be required for only one eye, it is important to distinguish clearly which eye is to be treated, using the traditional Latin identification, "oculus dexter" or "oculus sinister."

A colleague who had treated a patient in the hospital asked her to continue at home with the treatment that had been successful so far. Realizing that it might be a couple of days before the patient could get her prescription filled at a local pharmacy, he provided 10 tablets to cover the interim. So that the tablets would not be forgotten by the patient "on departure," he left written instructions that they were to be given to her "OD." As the patient was leaving, the nurse insisted that the physician intended all 10 tablets to be taken as "one dose," to which the patient first demurred and then acquiesced. Neither my colleague nor the nurse was present in the emergency department 4 hours later when their unconscious patient was brought in with a diagnosis that the ambulance crew had written as "drug OD."

WHY DOES IT MATTER?

"A desire to take medicine," as Osler[5] said, "is perhaps the great feature which distinguishes man from other animals." Today, that desire remains undiminished, but now it is coupled with the modern physician's equally strong desire to prescribe drugs that are much more potent than were the remedies available to Osler. The wrong dose or frequency of administration or drug interaction can result in disaster. Twenty years ago it was reported[4] that the number of drugs taken by patients during their hospital stay ranged from 5 to 31, and a decade ago it was estimated that 10 percent of patients suffered from the efforts of their physician to treat them.[2]

Patients and many physicians persist with the erroneous belief that there are such entities as totally safe drugs. There are not. But precise prescribing can make them safer and can go a long way to preventing mistakes and miscommunication. Write prescriptions clearly and precisely, and do not assume that your colleagues or patients will understand your imprecision or even interpret correctly your ambiguity.

REFERENCES

1. Burt, RAP: JAMA, 259:1330, 1988.
2. Davies, DM: *Textbook of Adverse Drug Reactions*. Oxford University Press, Oxford and New York, 1977, p 3.
3. Dunlop, DM: J Clin Pharmacol 7:184, 1967.
4. Lasagna, L: In Meyler, L and Peck HM (eds): Drug-induced Diseases. Exerpta Medica Foundation, Amsterdam, New York and London, 1965, p 1.
5. Osler, W: Science, New York 17:170, 1891.

SPECIAL DOSING CONSIDERATIONS*

For almost every drug there is an average dosing range. There are many common situations, however, when this average range can be either toxic or ineffective. The purpose of this section is to describe situations in which special dosing considerations must be made to assure a successful therapeutic outcome. The guidelines presented are general but should lead to a finer appreciation of individual dosing parameters. When you encounter these clinical situations, review the dose of drugs ordered and be sure that the necessary adjustments have been made.

THE PEDIATRIC PATIENT

The most obvious reason for adjusting dosages in pediatric patients is size. Most drug dosages for this population are given on a mg per kg body weight basis, or even more specifically on the basis of body surface area (BSA). Body surface area is determined by using a West or Body Surface Area Nomogram (p.l l). By drawing a straight line from the patient's height to the patient's weight, you will be able to read body surface area at the point wnere this line intersects the Body Surface Area line. Body surface area is expressed in square meters (m^2). The nomogram reflects the large range of sizes in this group, from the neonate and premature infant to the 12-year-old who is basically an adult in terms of drug absorption, distribution, metabolism, and excretion.

The neonate and the premature infant require additional adjustments besides those made on the basis of size. In this population, absorption following oral administration may be incomplete or altered due to changes in gastric pH or GI motility; distribution may be altered due to varying amounts of total body water; and metabolism and excretion may be delayed because liver and kidney function have not yet matured. Hepatic and renal maturation and weight changes may necessitate frequent dosage adjustments during the course of therapy and may have to be readjusted to reflect improved drug handling, even over several days, in the premature infant or neonate. In addition to pharmacokinetic variables, other considerations should be made. The route to administration chosen in pediatric patients often reflects the seriousness of the illness. The physician should consider the child's developmental level and ability to understand the situation. Medications that must be administered intravenously or by intramuscular injection may seem frightening to a young child or cause undo concern to the parents. The physician should allay these fears by educating the parents and child. Intramuscular or subcutaneous injection sites should be carefully chosen in this age group to prevent any possible nerve or tissue damage.

*From Deglin, JH and Vallerand, AH: *Davis's Drug Guide for Nurses.* FA Davis, Philadelphia, 1988, pp 5–11, with permission.

THE GERIATRIC PATIENT

In patients over age 60, the pharmacokinetic behavior of drugs changes. Drug absorption may be delayed secondary to diminished GI motility (from age or other drugs) or passive congestion of abdominal blood vessels, as seen in congestive heart failure. Distribution may be altered due to low plasma proteins, particularly in malnourished patients. Because plasma proteins are decreased, a larger proportion of free or unbound drug will result in an increase in drug action. This may result in the patient becoming toxic while receiving a standard dose of a drug. Metabolism performed by the liver and excretion handled by the kidneys are both slowed as part of the aging process and may cause prolonged and exaggerated drug action. Body composition also changes with age. There is an increase in fatty tissue and a decrease in skeletal muscle and total body water. Height and weight also usually decrease. A dosage of medication that was fine for the robust 50-year-old patient may be excessive in the same patient 20 years later.

An additional concern is that most elderly patients are already receiving numerous drugs. With increasing numbers of drugs being used, there is an increased risk of one drug negating, potentiating, or otherwise altering the effects of another drug (drug-drug interaction). In general, doses of most medications should be decreased in the geriatric population. Drugs of special concern are the digitalis glycosides, sedatives, hypnotics, oral anticoagulants, and antihypertensives.

Dosing regimens should be kept simple in this patient population, inasmuch as many of these patients are taking multiple drugs. Doses should be scheduled so that the patient's day is not interrupted numerous times to take medications. The use of fixed-dose combination drugs may help simplify dosing regimens. However, some of these combinations are more expensive than the individual components.

In explaining medication regimens to elderly patients, bear in mind that hearing deficits are common in this age group. Patients may find it embarrassing to disclose this information, and full compliance may be hindered.

THE OBSTETRICAL PATIENT

During pregnancy both the mother and the fetus must be considered. The placenta, once thought to be a protective barrier, is simply a membrane that is capable only of protecting the fetus from extremely large molecules. The placenta may transfer drugs to the fetus by both passive and active processes. The fetus is particularly vulnerable during two of the three stages of pregnancy: the first trimester and the last trimester. During the first trimester, the vital organs are being formed. Ingestion of drugs that cause harm (potential teratogens) during this stage of pregnancy may lead to fetal malformation or miscarriage. Unfortunately, this is the time when a woman is least likely to know that she is pregnant. Therefore, it is wise to inform all patients of childbearing age of this potential harm to an unborn child.

The possibility of medications altering sperm quality and quantity in potential fathers is also becoming an area of increasing concern. These considerations should be explained to patients who are trying to conceive. In the third trimester, the major concern is that drugs administered to the mother and transferred to the fetus may not be safely metabolized and excreted by the fetus. This is especially true of drugs administered near term. After the infant is delivered, he/she no longer has the placenta available to help with drug excretion.

There are situations in which, for the sake of the mother's health and to protect the fetus, drug administration is required throughout pregnancy. Two examples of this are the epileptic patient and the hypertensive patient. In these circumstances, the safest drug in the smallest possible doses is chosen. Because of changes in the behavior of drugs that may occur throughout pregnancy, dosage adjustments may be required during the progression of pregnancy and after delivery.

RENAL FUNCTION

The kidneys are the major organs of drug elimination. Some drugs are excreted only after being metabolized or biotransformed by the liver. Others may be eliminated unchanged by the kidneys. The premature infant has immature renal function. Elderly patients have an age-related decrease in renal function. In order to make dosage adjustments in patients with renal dysfunction, you must know the degree of renal impairment in the individual patient and the percentage of drug that is eliminated by the kidneys. The degree of renal function can be quantitated by laboratory testing, most commonly by the creatinine clearance. The percentage of each drug excreted by the kidneys can be determined from references on pharmacokinetics. In addition, the dosage frequently can be optimized by measuring blood levels of the drug in the individual patient and making any further necessary changes. Two types of drugs for which this type of dosage adjustment are commonly used are digoxin and the aminoglycoside antibiotics (amikacin, gentamicin, tobramycin).

LIVER DISEASE

The liver is the major organ for metabolism of drugs. For most drugs, this is an inactivation step. Most inactive metabolites are subsequently excreted by the kidneys. The conversion process usually changes the drug from a relatively lipid- or fat-soluble compound to a more water-soluble substance. Liver function is not as easily quantified as renal function, therefore it is difficult to predict the correct dosage for a patient with liver dysfunction based on laboratory tests alone. In addition, it appears that only a minimal level of liver function may be required for complete drug metabolism.

A patient who is severely jaundiced or has very low serum proteins (particularly albumin) may be expected to have some problems metabolizing drugs. Chronic alcoholic patients are at risk for developing this type of situation. In advanced liver disease, drug absorption may also be impaired secondary to portal vascular congestion. Examples of drugs that should be carefully dosed in patients with liver disease include theophylline and sedatives, which are metabolized by the liver. Some drugs require the liver for activation (such as sulindac or cyclophosphamide) and should be avoided in patients with severely compromised liver function.

CONGESTIVE HEART FAILURE

Patients with clinical congestive heart failure also require dosage modifications. In these patients, drug absorption may be impaired due to passive congestion of blood vessels feeding the GI tract. This same passive congestion slows drug delivery to the liver and delays metabolism. In addition, renal function may be compromised, leading to delayed elimination and prolonged drug action. Many patients who have congestive heart failure are already in a special dosing category because of their age. Dosages of drugs that are mainly metabolized by the liver or mainly excreted by the kidneys should be decreased in patients with apparent congestive heart failure.

OBESITY

In most situations, drug dosing is based on total weight. Some drugs selectively penetrate fatty tissues. If the drug is known to not penetrate fatty tissues and the patient is obese, dosage should be determined by ideal body weight or estimated lean body mass. These quantities may be determined from tables of desirable weights or may be estimated using formulas for lean body mass when the patient's height and weight are known. If this type of adjustment is not made, considerable toxicity may result.

DELIVERY TO SITES OF ACTION

In order to have a successful therapeutic outcome, the drug must reach its intended site of action. Under the most desirable of conditions, the drug will have only a minimal effect on other tissues or body systems. A good example is drugs that are applied topically for skin conditions and are only minimally absorbed. Sometimes unusual routes of administration must be used to guarantee the presence of drug at the intended site of response. For example, in patients with bacterial meningitis, administering drugs parenterally may not produce high enough levels in the cerebrospinal fluid. Intrathecal administration may be required in addition to parenteral therapy. The eye also presents a barrier that is relatively impermeable to many drugs. To overcome this, local instillation or injection may be required.

In some cases, local absorption may not occur and therefore the desired systemic effect will not occur. In patients with shock or poor tissue perfusion due to other causes, drugs may not be absorbed into systemic circulation from subcutaneous sites.

When considering the route of administration, remember where the drug is intended to have its primary action. In order to achieve its maximal effect it must be delivered to its intended site of action.

DRUG INTERACTIONS

The presence of other drugs may necessitate dosage adjustments. Drugs, such as warfarin and phenytoin, that are highly bound to plasma proteins may be displaced by other highly protein-bound drugs. When this phenomenon occurs, the drug that has been displaced exhibits an increase in its activity because it is the free, or unbound, drug that is active.

Some agents decrease the ability of the liver to metabolize other drugs. Drugs that are capable of doing this include cimetidine and chloramphenicol. Concurrently administered drugs that are highly metabolized by the liver may need to be administered in decreased dosages. Other agents, such as phenobarbital, other barbiturates, and rifampin, are capable of stimulating (inducing) the liver to metabolize drugs more rapidly, requiring larger doses to be administered.

Drugs that significantly alter urine pH can affect excretion of other drugs for which the excretory process is pH dependent. Alkalinizing the urine will hasten the excretion of acidic drugs. Acidification of the urine will enhance reabsorption of acidic drugs, prolonging and enhancing drug action. In the reverse situation, drugs that acidify the urine will hasten the excretion of alkaline drugs.

Some drugs compete with other drugs for enzyme systems. Allopurinol inhibits the enzyme that is involved in uric acid production, but it also inhibits the metabolism (inactivation) of 6-mercaptopurine, greatly increasing its toxicity. The dosage of mercaptopurine needs to be significantly reduced when coadministered with allopurinol.

DOSAGE FORMS

The physician will frequently encounter problems that relate to the dosage form itself. Some medications may not be commercially available in liquid or chewable dosage forms. The pharmacist may have to compound such dosage forms for an individual patient. It may be necessary to disguise the taste or appearance of a medication in food or a beverage in order for the patient to fully comply with a given regimen. Finally, some dosage forms, such as aerosol inhalers, may not be suitable for very young patients because their use requires cooperation beyond the patient's age level.

Before altering dosage forms (crushing tablets or opening capsules) check to be sure that the effect of the drug won't be altered by doing so. In general, extended or prolonged release dosage forms should not be crushed, nor should capsules containing beads of medication opened. Altering these dosage forms may shorten and intensify their intended action. Enteric coated tablets, which may appear to be sugar-coated or candy-coated, also should not be crushed. This coating is designed to protect the stomach from the irritating effects of these drugs. Crushing them will expose the stomach lining to these agents and increase GI irritation. If a dosage form needs to be crushed, it should be ingested right away. A glass of water should be taken prior to administration of powders or crushed tablets to wet the esophagus and prevent the material from sticking to upper GI mucosal surfaces.

ENVIRONMENTAL FACTORS

Cigarette smoke is capable of inducing liver enzymes to metabolize drugs more rapidly. Patients who smoke may need larger doses of liver-metabolized drugs to compensate for this. Patients who are passively exposed to cigarette smoke may also exhibit otherwise unexplained needs for larger doses of medications.

NUTRITIONAL FACTORS

Certain foods can alter the dosing requirement for some medications. Dietary calcium found in high concentrations in dairy products combines with tetracycline and prevents its absorption. Many antibiotics are absorbed better if taken when the stomach is empty. Large doses of antacid will decrease the effect of aspirin. Foods that are high in pyridoxine (vitamin B_6) can negate the antiparkinson effect of levodopa (this is counteracted with coadministration of carbidopa). Foods that are capable of altering urine pH may affect the excretion patterns of medications, either enhancing or diminishing their effectiveness. There are no general guidelines for nutritional factors. It is prudent to check if these problems exist or if they may explain therapeutic failures and to make the necessary dosage adjustments.

SUMMARY

The average dosing range for drugs is intended for an average patient. However, every patient is an individual with specific drug-handling capabilities. Taking into account these special dosing considerations allows the planning of an individualized drug regimen that will result in a desired therapuetic outcome while minimizing the risk of toxicity.

NOMOGRAM*

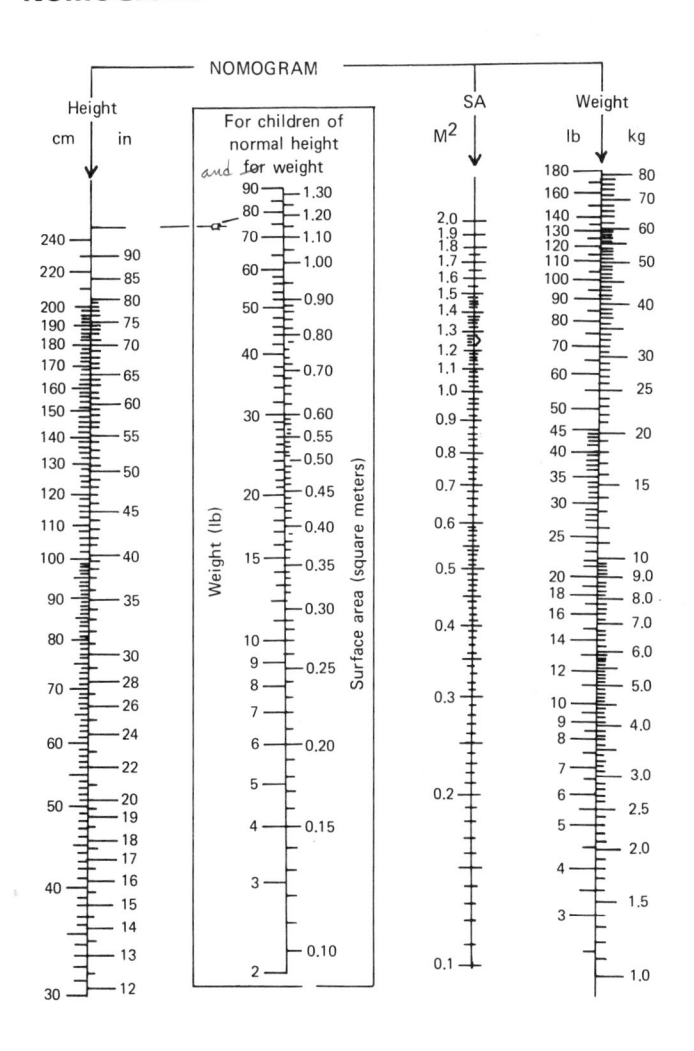

*From Deglin, JH and Vallerand, AH: *Davis's Drug Guide for Nurses*. FA Davis, Philadelphia, 1988, p 707, with permission.

SCHEDULES OF CONTROLLED DRUGS*

Schedule I: Drugs in this class are not available for legitimate use for any purposes other than investigative ones. Clearance from the FDA is required before these drugs (for example, LSD and marijuana) can be legally obtained.

Schedule II: Drugs in this class have high abuse potentials that may lead to severe psychologic or physical dependence or both. No telephoned prescriptions will be filled. Each refill must be reordered with a new prescription.

Examples of Schedule II Drugs:

amphetamine	methadone
codeine	methylphenidate
dextroamphetamine	morphine
droperidol with fentanyl	oxycodone
hydromorphone	pentobarbital
meperidine	secobarbital

For hospitalized patients, you must rewrite routine orders for drugs in schedules III, IV, and V every 7 days and PRN orders every 72 hours. You must sign phone orders within 48 hours.

Schedule III: Drugs in this class have a lower abuse potential than those in either schedule I or schedule II. These prescriptions can be filled by telephone. They must be rewritten every 6 months or after 5 refills, whichever comes first.

Example of Schedule III Drugs:
codeine (when combined with selected drugs)

Schedule IV: This schedule is similar to schedule III, except for the penalties for illegal possession.

Examples of Schedule IV Drugs:

alprazolam	midazolam
chloral hydrate	oxazepam
chlordiazepoxide	pemoline
clonazepam	pentazocine
clorazepate	phenobarbital
diazepam	prazepam
flurazepam	propoxyphene
lorazepam	temazepam
meprobamate	triazolam

---

*Adapted from Mathewson, M: *Pharmacotherapeutics: A Nursing Process Approach.* FA Davis, Philadelphia, 1986, with permission.

Schedule V: According to federal law, this class of drugs has a low abuse potential, does not require a prescription, and is sold over the counter. Most states, however, have a stricter ruling that requires prescriptions and the same refill regulations as schedules III and IV.

Examples of Schedule V Drugs:

buprenorphine
codeine (cough preparations)
diphenoxylate with atropine
paregoric

COMMONLY USED ABBREVIATIONS

ac	before meals
AD	right ear
AS	left ear
AU	both ears
bid	two times a day
$\bar{c}$	with
cap	capsule
D5W	5% dextrose in water
D10W	10% dextrose in water
Gm or g	gram(s)
gr	grain(s)
gtt	drop(s)
h or hr	hour(s)
hs	hour of sleep (bed time)
IM	intramuscular
Inhal or Inhaln	inhalation
I & O	intake and output
IT	intrathecal
IV	intravenous
L	liter
LR	lactated Ringer's solution
M	minim
MAO	monoamine oxidase
mcg	microgram(s)
mg	milligram(s)
ml	milliliter(s)
NS	normal saline (0.9% NaCL)
NSAI	nonsteroidal anti-inflammatory agent(s)
OD	right eye
Oint	ointment
Ophth	ophthalmic
OS	left eye
OU	both eyes
oz	ounce(s)
pc	after meals
PO	by mouth, orally
prn	when required
q	every
qd	every day
qh	every hour
qod	every other day
qwk	every week
q2h	every 2 hours
q3h	every 3 hours
q4h	every 4 hours
qid	four times a day
qs	as much as is required
Rect	rectally

s̄	without
SC	subcutaneous
SL	sublingual
SR	sustained release
s̄s̄	one half
stat	immediately
supp	suppository
tab	tablet
Tbs	tablespoon(s)
tid	three times a day
Top	topically
tsp	teaspoon(s)

100 MOST FREQUENTLY PRESCRIBED HOSPITAL DRUGS BY PHARMACOLOGIC CLASS

Antacids
Aluminum hydroxide, aluminum carbonate, magaldrate, magnesium hydroxide and aluminum hydroxide, 23
Calcium carbonate, 34
Milk of magnesia, 87
Sodium bicarbonate, 118

Antianemic
Ferrous salts, 59

Antiarrhythmics
Digoxin, 50
Lidocaine, 78
Phenytoin, 103
Procainamide, 110
Propranolol, 112
Quinidine, 114
Verapamil, 132

Antibiotics
Carbapenems:
  Imipenem/Cilastatin, 70
Aminoglycosides:
  Gentamicin, 63
Cephalosporins:
  Cefazolin, 37
  Cefoxitin, 38
  Ceftriaxone, 39
Penicillins:
  Ampicillin, 28
  Azlocillin, 32
  Nafcillin, 90
  Penicillin G or V, 99
Sulfonamides:
  Sulfasalazine, 122
  Sulfisoxazole, 123
Tetracyclines:
  Tetracycline, 126
Miscellaneous:
  Clindamycin, 43
  Erythromycin, 58
  Nitrofurantoin, 92
  Norfloxacin, 96
  Trimethoprim-Sulfamethoxazole, 130
  Vancomycin, 131

Anticoagulants
Heparin, 65
Warfarin, 135

Anticonvulsants
Carbamazepine, 36
Diazepam, 49
Phenobarbital, 101
Phenytoin, 103

Antidepressants
Amitriptyline, 25
Trazodone, 128

Antidiarrheal
Diphenoxylate with atropine, 54

Antiemetics
Metoclopramide, 86
Prochlorperazine, 111

Antifungals
Amphotericin B, 27
Nystatin, 97

Antigout Agents
Allopurinol, 22
Probenecid, 109

Antihistamine
Diphenhydramine, 53

Antihypertensive Agents
Beta-adrenoceptor antagonists:
  Atenolol, 31
  Labetolol, 75
  Propranolol, 112
α_1- and α_2-adrenoceptor agonists:
  Clonidine, 44
  α-Methyldopa, 85
ACE inhibitors:
  Captopril, 35
Vasodilators:
  Hydralazine, 66
  Minoxidil, 88
  Nitroprusside, 95
  Prazosin, 106

Diuretics:
  Furosemide, 61
  Hydrochlorothiazide, 67

Antimanic Agent
Lithium, 79

Antineoplastics
Alkylating agents:
  Cyclophosphamide, 45
Antitumor antibiotics:
  Doxorubicin, 57
Antimetabolites:
  Fluorouracil, 60
  Methotrexate, 83
Hormonal agents:
  Tamoxifen, 124
Vinca alkaloids:
  Vinblastine, 133
  Vincristine, 134

Antiparkinson Agents
Diphenhydramine, 53
Levodopa/Carbidopa, 76

Antiplatelet Agent
Aspirin, 29

Antipsychotics
Chlorpromazine, 40
Haloperidol, 64
Prochlorperazine, 111

Antipyretics
Acetaminophen, 21
Aspirin, 29

Antituberculars
Isoniazid, 73
Rifampin, 117

Antitussive
Diphenhydramine, 53

Antiulcer Agents
Aluminum hydroxide, aluminum carbonate, magaldrate, magnesium hydroxide and aluminum hydroxide, 23
Cimetidine, 42
Ranitidine, 116
Sucralfate, 121

Beta-Adrenoceptor Antagonists
Atenolol, 31
Labetolol, 75
Propranolol, 112

Bronchodilators
Metaproterenol, 81
Terbutaline, 125
Theophylline, 127

Calcium Channel Antagonists
Diltiazem, 51
Nifedipine, 91
Verapamil, 132

Cardiac Glycoside
Digoxin, 50

Coronary Vasodilators
Diltiazem, 52
Isosorbide dinitrate, 74
Nifedipine, 91
Nitroglycerin, 93
Verapamil, 132

Diuretics
Loop diuretics:
  Furosemide, 61
Potassium-sparing diuretics:
  Amiloride, 24
  Spironolactone, 120
  Triamterene, 129
Thiazide diuretics:
  Hydrochlorothiazide, 67

Electrolytes/Electrolyte Modifiers
Alkalinizer:
  Sodium bicarbonate, 118
Calcium salts:
  Calcium carbonate, 34
Hypophosphatemic
  Aluminum hydroxide, 23
Magnesium salts
  Magnesium hydroxide, 23
Potassium exchange resin
  Sodium polystyrene sulfonate, 119
Potassium salts
  Potassium chloride, 105

Glucocorticoids
Intermediate-acting:
  Prednisone, 107
Long-acting:
  Dexamethasone, 47

H$_2$-Receptor Antagonists
Cimetidine, 42
Ranitidine, 116

Hormones
Insulin, 72
Levothyroxine, 77

Immunosuppressants
Cyclophosphamide, 45
Cyclosporine, 46
Methotrexate, 83

Inotropic Agents
Digoxin, 50
Dopamine, 56

Laxatives
Bisacodyl, 33
Docusate, 55
Milk of magnesia, 87

Nonnarcotic Analgesics
Nonsteroidal anti-inflammatory drugs:
  Aspirin, 29
  Ibuprofen, 69
  Indomethacin, 71
Miscellaneous anti-inflammatory drugs:
  Acetaminophen, 21

Opioid Analgesics
Meperidine, 80
Methadone, 82
Morphine sulfate, 89
Oxycodone, 98

Sedative/Hypnotics
Diazepam, 49
Phenobarbital, 101

Skeletal Muscle Relaxant
Diazepam, 49

Vasopressor
Dopamine, 56

100 MOST FREQUENTLY PRESCRIBED HOSPITAL DRUGS BY GENERIC NAME

Acetaminophen, 21
Allopurinol, 22
Aluminum hydroxide, aluminum carbonate, magaldrate, magnesium hydroxide and aluminum hydroxide, 23
Amiloride, 24
Amitriptyline, 25
Amphotericin B, 27
Ampicillin, 28
Aspirin, 29
Atenolol, 31
Azlocillin, 32
Bisacodyl, 33
Calcium carbonate, 34
Captopril, 35
Carbamazepine, 36
Cefazolin, 37
Cefoxitin, 38
Ceftriaxone, 39
Chlorpromazine, 40
Cimetidine, 42
Clindamycin, 43
Clonidine, 44
Cyclophosphamide, 45
Cyclosporine, 46
Dexamethasone, 47
Diazepam, 49
Digoxin, 50
Diltiazem, 52
Diphenhydramine, 53
Diphenoxylate with atropine, 54
Docusate, 55
Dopamine, 56
Doxorubicin, 57
Erythromycin, 58
Ferrous salts, 59
Fluorouracil, 60
Furosemide, 61
Gentamicin, 63
Haloperidol, 64
Heparin, 65
Hydralazine, 66
Hydrochlorothiazide, 67
Ibuprofen, 69
Imipenem/Cilastatin, 70
Indomethacin, 71

Insulin, 72
Isoniazid, 73
Isosorbide dinitrate, 74
Labetolol, 75
Levodopa/Carbidopa, 76
Levothyroxine, 77
Lidocaine, 78
Lithium, 79
Meperidine, 80
Metaproterenol, 81
Methadone, 82
Methotrexate, 83
α-Methyldopa, 85
Metoclopramide, 86
Milk of magnesia, 87
Minoxidil, 88
Morphine sulfate, 89
Nafcillin, 90
Nifedipine, 91
Nitrofurantoin, 92
Nitroglycerin, 93
Nitroprusside, 95
Norfloxacin, 96
Nystatin, 97
Oxycodone, 98
Penicillin G or V, 99
Phenobarbital, 101
Phenytoin, 103
Potassium chloride, 105
Prazosin, 106
Prednisone, 107
Probenecid, 109
Procainamide, 110
Prochlorperazine, 111
Propranolol, 112
Quinidine, 114
Ranitidine, 116
Rifampin, 117
Sodium bicarbonate, 118
Sodium polystyrene sulfonate, 119
Spironolactone, 120
Sucralfate, 121
Sulfasalazine, 122
Sulfisoxazole, 123
Tamoxifen, 124
Terbutaline, 125

Tetracycline, 126
Theophylline, 127
Trazodone, 128
Triamterene, 129
Trimethoprim-Sulfamethoxazole, 130
Vancomycin, 131
Verapamil, 132
Vinblastine, 133
Vincristine, 134
Warfarin, 135

ACETAMINOPHEN (PARACETAMOL) (Anacin-3, Datril, Panadol, Tempra, Tylenol)

Pharmacologic Class: Nonnarcotic analgesic, antipyretic.

Mechanism of Action: Mechanism is unclear. It has a direct action on the hypothalamic heat-regulating center. CNS inhibition of prostaglandin synthesis.

Indication: Mild to moderate pain and fever.

Route of Excretion: Extensively metabolized by the liver. Metabolites excreted by the kidney.

Dosage (oral and rectal):
Adult: 650–1000 mg q 4–6 hr. Do not exceed 4000 mg/24 hr.
Pediatric: Approximately 10 mg/kg/dose. Do not exceed 5 doses/day.

11–12 yr	480 mg q 4–6 hr prn
9–10 yr	400 mg q 4–6 hr prn
6– 8 yr	320 mg q 4–6 hr prn
4– 5 yr	240 mg q 4–6 hr prn
2– 3 yr	160 mg q 4–6 hr prn
1– 2 yr	120 mg q 4–6 hr prn
4–12 mos	80 mg q 4–6 hr prn
0– 3 mos	40 mg q 4–6 hr prn

Adverse Reactions: Side effects rare at recommended doses.

Overdosage: (>10 g) Acetaminophen serum levels >300 mcg/ml 4 hr after ingestion with severe hepatic damage, >200–300 mcg/ml with mild to severe liver toxicity. Symptoms (1–6 days): Nausea, vomiting, hepatotoxicity, pancytopenia, coma, death. Treatment: emesis, lavage, oral N-acetylcysteine.

Precautions:
Use cautiously in patients with impaired hepatic function.
Do not use >2.6 g/day chronically. Chronic high-dose ingestion may cause renal papillary necrosis, hepatic damage.

Contraindication: Hypersensitivity to acetaminophen.

Drug Interactions:
Barbiturates enhance metabolism of acetaminophen.
Activated charcoal reduces absorption of acetaminophen.
May potentiate salicylate renal toxicity with chronic high-dose use.

Monitor: Temperature, pain relief.

ALLOPURINOL (Zyloprim)

Pharmacologic Class: Antigout agent.

Mechanism of Action: Allopurinol and its active metabolic, oxypurinol, inhibit the synthesis of uric acid by inhibition of xanthine oxidase.

Indications:
Prevention of gouty arthritis and nephropathy.
Prevention of hyperuricemia in polycythemia vera, myeloid metaplasia, in patients receiving chemotherapy or radiation for leukemias and lymphomas.
Prevention of recurrent calcium oxalate calculi.

Route of Excretion: 20% Hepatic, allopurinol is metabolized to oxypurinol. Both allopurinol and oxypurinol are renally eliminated.

Dosage:
Adult: 100–800 mg/d, average 300 mg/d.
Pediatric (6–10yr): 300 mg; (<6 yr) 150 mg.
Renal Failure: Creatinine clearance (10–20 ml/min) 200 mg/d; (<10 ml/min) 100 mg q 24–48 hr.

Adverse Reactions: Maculopapular skin rash, Stevens-Johnson syndrome, hypersensitivity, bone marrow depression, nausea, vomiting, diarrhea, hepatotoxicity, drowsiness, interstitial nephritis.

Contraindications: Hypersensitivity, pregnancy, lactation.

Precautions: Allopurinol may precipitate acute gouty attacks. Consider prophylactic colchicine, increase allopurinol dose slowly.

Drug Interactions:
Allopurinol inhibits metabolism of azathioprine and 6-mercaptopurine (6MP) azathioprine/6 MP. Reduce dose to $1/4$–$1/3$ of usual dose.
Increased incidence of skin rash in patients treated concomitantly with allopurinol and ampicillin or amoxicillin.
Increased incidence of hypersensitivity reactions in patients receiving thiazide diutetics concurrently with allopurinol.
Allopurinol may inhibit metabolism of oral anticoagulants. Recheck PT.
Increased risk of hypoglycemia in patients treated with chlorpropamide due to decreased renal excretion caused by allopurinol.
Uricosuric agents increase the clearance of oxypurinol.

Monitor: Serum uric acid. Check blood counts, liver and kidney functions.

ALUMINUM HYDROXIDE (Alternagel, Alucaps, Alutabs, Amphogel)
ALUMINUM CARBONATE (Basaljel)
MAGALDRATE (Riopan)
MAGNESIUM HYDROXIDE AND ALUMINUM HYDROXIDE
(Gelusil, Maalox, Mylanta, WinGel)

Pharmacologic Class: Nonsystemic antacid.

Mechanism of Action: Neutralizes or reduces gastric acidity. Aluminum-containing antacids form insoluble aluminum phosphate which aids in fecal excretion of phosphate in patients with renal failure.

Indications:
Treatment of peptic ulcers.
Prophylaxis of GI bleeding.
Symptomatic relief of reflux esophagitis and indigestion.
Aluminum antacids also used for hyperphosphatemia in renal failure.

Dosage:
Depends on concentration and acid-neutralizing capacity of product chosen. Generally 5–30 ml or 1 to 2 tablets 1 and 3 hr after meals and at bedtime.
For hyperphosphatemia, aluminum antacids 5–30 ml or 1–4 tablets after meals.

Adverse Reactions: Constipation, nausea, and vomiting (aluminum salts); **diarrhea** (magnesium salts); hypophosphatemia, hypermagnesemia (magnesium salts); dialysis dementia and osteomalacia (aluminum salts).

Precautions: Avoid use of magnesium salts in renal failure.

Drug Interactions:
Antacids may decrease the absorption of anticholinergics, iron salts, isoniazid, phenothiazines, and tetracycline.
Aluminum hydroxide may decrease the absorption of corticosteroids, digoxin, isoniazid, phenytoin, quinidine, and warfarin.

Monitor: Bowel movements, stool guaiac, symptomatic relief, magnesium, phosphate.

AMILORIDE (Midamor)

Pharmacologic Class: Potassium-sparing diuretic.

Mechanism of action: Directly inhibits sodium reabsorption and potassium secretion at the renal distal tubule. May inhibit sodium-potassium–ATPase.

Indications:
Prevent or treat hypokalemia.
Use in combination with other agents to treat edema or hypertension.

Pharmacodynamics: Onset 2 hr, peak 6–10 hr, duration 24 hr.

Route of Excretion: Renal 50%. Feces 40% (unabsorbed drug).

Dosage: 5–20 mg orally daily.

Side Effects: Hyperkalemia, anorexia, **headache, nausea,** vomiting, **diarrhea.**

Precautions: Increased risk of hyperkalemia in patients with diabetes mellitus and acidosis.

Contraindications:
Hypersensitivity or renal impairment, hyperkalemia, patients treated with concomitant potassium supplements or other potassium-sparing diuretics (spironolactone or triamterene).
Avoid in pregnant women or nursing mothers.

Drug Interactions:
Additive hypotension with other antihypertensive agents.
Increased risk of hyperkalemia in patients treated concomitantly with captopril, enalapril, lisinopril, triamterene, spironolactone, or potassium supplements.
Increased risk of lithium toxicity due to reduction of lithium's renal clearance by amiloride.

Monitor: Serum electrolytes (Na^+, K^+, Cl^-, HCO_3^-), BUN, creatinine, weight, blood pressure.

AMITRIPTYLINE (Elavil, Endep)
(Other tricyclics: imipramine, desipramine, doxepin, nortriptyline, protriptyline)

Pharmacologic Class: Tertiary amine, tricyclic antidepressant.

Mechanism of Action: Unclear. May block neurotransmitter reuptake of norepinephrine or serotonin. May decrease number of presynaptic alpha$_2$ receptors. Also sedative and anticholinergic effects. Antidepressant effect may take days to weeks.

Indication:
Treatment of depression.
Also used for cluster and migraine headaches.

Pharmacodynamics:

Peak Plasma	Half-life	Onset	Therapeutic Plasma
2–4 hr	31–46 hr	2–4 wk	>200 ng/ml

Route of Excretion: Metabolized by liver to form active metabolite, nortriptyline.

Dosage:
po 25–300 mg/d. May administer hs or in 3 divided doses.
IM 20–30 mg qid.

Adverse Reactions: Sedation, confusion, orthostatic hypotension, anticholinergic effects **(dry mouth, blurred vision, urinary retention, tachycardia, constipation),** arrhythmias, allergic skin reactions, blood dyscrasias, photosensitivity, sleep disturbances, tremors, gynecomastia.

Precautions: Use cautiously in elderly and patients with cardiovascular disease, prostatic hypertrophy, and seizure disorders.

Contraindications:
Hypersensitivity; narrow-angle glaucoma; avoid in pregnancy and lactation (crosses placenta and excreted in breast milk).
Do not use concomitantly with MAO inhibitors.

Drug Interactions:
Concomitant use of tricyclics with MAO inhibitors may cause hyperpyretic crises, severe seizures, hypertensive episodes, and death.
Tricyclics antagonize antihypertensive effect of guanethidine and clonidine.
Additive CNS depression when used in combination with alcohol, antihistamines, barbiturates, benzodiazepines, narcotics, and sedative/hypnotic agents.
Decreased blood levels of tricyclics due to enhanced metabolism by barbiturates, smoking.
Increased blood levels of tricyclics due to impaired metabolism by cimetidine, methylphenidate, phenothiazines, oral contraceptives.

Tricyclics may enhance pressor response of epinephrine, norepinephrine, and phenylephrine.

Do not use concomitantly with metrizamide. Discontinue tricyclics 2 days before to 1 day after myelography.

Additive atropine-like effects when used in combination with anticholinergic agents.

Monitor: Plasma levels, symptomatic response to TCA (2–4 wk after initiation); postural blood pressure, heart rate; anticholinergic and sedative effects.

AMPHOTERICIN B (Fungizone)

Pharmacologic Class: Antifungal agent.

Mechanism of Action: Binds to fungal cell membrane and causes a change in membrane permeability.

Indication:
Treatment of serious fungal infections, including aspergillosis, blastomycosis, disseminated candidiasis, coccidiomycosis, cryptococcosis, histoplasmosis, mucormycosis, and sporotrichosis.
Topical preparation for cutaneous and mucocutaneous candidal infections.

Route of Excretion: Unknown. Only 2–5% excreted in unchanged form by kidneys. No dosage alteration required in patients with impaired renal function.

Dosage:
Administer 1 mg test dose. Infuse dose over 6 hr at concentration of 100 mcg/ml. Initiate therapy with 0.25 mg/kg/d, increase dose as tolerated up to 1 mg/kg/d or 1.5 mg/kg every other day.
Applied topically (cream, lotion, ointment) 2–4 times daily.

Adverse Reactions: Fever, shaking chills, headache, generalized pain; phlebitis, anorexia, **nausea,** vomiting, diarrhea, dyspepsia; **hypokalemia,** hypomagnesemia, renal tubular acidosis, azotemia **(nephrotoxicity** may be irreversible at total dose >5 g), normochromic normocytic anemia. Adverse reactions may be lessened by pretreatment with antipyretics, antihistamines, corticosteroids, and/or meperidine.

Precautions:
Administer in hospital or under close medical supervision.
If liver function or renal tests (BUN$>$40, Cr $>$3) become abnormal, discontinue therapy or reduce dose until function improves.

Contraindication: Hypersensitivity.

Drug Interactions:
Additive nephrotoxicity with nephrotoxic antibiotics (.e.g, aminoglycosides), antineoplastics (cisplatin), and cyclosporine. Corticosteroids and diuretics may increase risk of hypokalemia when used with amphotericin B.
Hypokalemia due to amphotericin B may potentiate effect of skeletal muscle relaxants and digitalis glycosides.

Monitor: Serum potassium, creatinine, bicarbonate, magnesium; BUN; temperature, hemoglobin.

AMPICILLIN (Amcill, Omnipen, Polycillin, Principen)

(Other antibiotics with similar spectrum of action: bacampicillin, amoxicillin)

Pharmacologic Class: Antibiotic—penicillin.

Mechanism of Action: Bactericidal effect due to inhibition of synthesis of cell wall mucopeptide.

Indications: Infections caused by susceptible organisms: *E. coli, H influenzae, Enterococci, Streptococci, Pneumococci, N. Gonorrhoeae, N. meningitidis, Proteus mirabilis, Shigella, Salmonella.*

Pharmacokinetics: Absorption (30–50%), peak 1.5–2.0 hr. Variable metabolism by liver depending on route of administration; % excreted renally, unchanged: 25–60% after oral; 50–90% after parenteral; half-life 0.8–1.5 hr.

Dosage:
Dosage reduction may be needed in severe renal disease.
Oral
  Pediatric (<20 kg): 50–100 mg/kg/d in 3–4 divided doses.
  Adult: 250–500 mg q 6 hr.
IV/IM
  Pediatric (>40 kg): 25–50 mg/kg/d in 3–4 divided doses.
  Adult: 1–12 g/d.

Adverse Reactions: Rash, diarrhea, nausea, vomiting; superinfection; fever; anaphylaxis, blood dyscrasias, interstitial nephritis, seizures (with excessive doses).

Contraindication: Hypersensitivity to penicillins.

Precautions:
Increased incidence of rash in patients with lymphocytic leukemia and mononucleosis, and concomitant treatment with allopurinol.
Cross-sensitivity between penicillins and cephalosporins.

Drug Interactions:
Probenicid decreases renal excretion causing increased blood levels.
Allopurinol use may increase risk of ampicillin skin rashes.
Ampicillin may decrease effectiveness of oral contraceptives.

Monitor: Temperature, WBC, culture and sensitivity.

ASPIRIN (Acetylsalicylic acid, ASA, Bayer, Ecotrin)

Pharmacologic Class: Nonnarcotic analgesic, nonsteroidal anti-inflammatory drug, antipyretic, antiplatelet agent.

Mechanism of Action: Inhibition of prostaglandin production by inactivating cyclo-oxygenase, causing decreased inflammation and platelet aggregation.

Indications:
Fever.
Mild to moderate pain.
Rheumatoid arthritis.
Prevention of transient ischemia attacks in men.
Myocardial infarction.

Pharmacokinetics: Absorption: Salicylates are well absorbed, although some enteric coated products may be erratically absorbed. Rectal administration results in slower absorption. Anti-inflammatory therapeutic concentrations 15–30 mg %.

Metabolism/Excretion: Half-life 15–20 minutes; at anti-inflammatory doses half-life increases to 6–12 hours. Extensively metabolized by liver. 2–3% excreted unchanged, inactive metabolites are renally excreted.

Dosage:

	Adult	**Pediatric**
Analgesic/antipyretic	325–650 mg q 4 hr prn	65 mg/kg/d in 4–6 divided doses
Anti-inflammatory	2.6–5.2 g/d in divided doses	90–130 mg/kg/d in divided doses

Prevent TIAs: 1300 mg/d in 2–4 divided doses.
Prevent MI: 325 mg q other day or daily.

Adverse Reactions: Anorexia, **nausea**, vomiting, **dyspepsia, epigastric distress**, GI bleeding, iron-deficiency anemia, allergy, anaphylactic reaction; salicylism: mild—tinnitus, nausea, vomiting, diarrhea, confusion, hearing loss; serious—hyperventilation, asterixis, convulsions, metabolic acidosis, renal failure, coma, cardiovascular collapse.

Contraindications: Hypersensitivity to salicylates, active peptic ulcer disease, hemophilia.

Precautions:
Use cautiously in patients with asthma, nasal polyps, rhinitis, history of GI ulcers, bleeding tendencies, severe anemia, or severe renal or hepatic disease; may need to order buffered or enteric coated tablets for patients at risk for gastritis.
May cause Reye's syndrome in children or adolescents with chickenpox or flu.

Drug Interactions:
Salicylates may potentiate effect of oral anticoagulants, oral hypoglycemics, and methotrexate.

Salicylates may antagonize effects of spironolactone, uricosuric agents (sulfinpyrazone, probenecid, phenylbutazone, oxyphenbutazone).

Glucocorticoids, sodium bicarbonate (at dose to alkalinize urine) may decrease serum salicylate levels.

Acetazolamide may worsen salicylate intoxication.

Ethanol may increase GI bleeding produced by salicylates.

Antacids may slow absorption.

Aspirin interferes with action of furosemide-like diuretics.

Monitor: Temperature, symptomatic relief, therapeutic anti-inflammatory serum concentrations 15–30 mg %, stool for occult blood.

ATENOLOL (Tenormin)
(Other selective beta adrenoceptor antagonists: metoprolol, acebutolol)

Pharmacologic Class: Selective beta adrenoceptor antagonist; antihypertensive.

Mechanism of Action: Blocks beta$_1$ (myocardial) adrenergic receptors, not usually beta$_2$ (pulmonary, vascular, uterine) receptors at therapeutic doses. Therapeutic effects include decreased heart rate, depressed AV conduction, decreased blood pressure, decreased cardiac output.

Indications:
Hypertension.
Angina pectoris.

Pharmacokinetics:
Incompletely absorbed (40–60%).
Absorbed drug excreted unchanged by kidney.
Does not significantly cross blood-brain barrier.
No direct correlation between dose or plasma level and therapeutic effect.

Dosage: 50–100 mg daily, decrease dose with renal failure.

Adverse Reactions: Fatigue, weakness, depression, dizziness; **bradycardia,** congestive heart failure, hypotension, pulmonary edema, bronchospasm, rhinitis; impotence; peripheral vascular insufficiency.

Contraindications: Sinus bradycardia or greater-than-first-degree heart block, uncompensated congestive heart failure, cardiogenic shock, pregnancy.

Precautions:
Abrupt discontinuation associated with exacerbation of angina, MI, and arrhythmias. Reduce gradually over 1–2 weeks.
Use cautiously in patients with asthma and emphysema.
Beta blockers may mask symptoms of acute hypoglycemia and thyrotoxicosis.

Drug Interactions:
General anesthesia, nifedipine, IV phenytoin, IV verapamil may have additive myocardial depressant effect.
Additive bradycardia with digitalis glycosides.
Additive decreased blood pressure with antihypertensive agents.
Ampicillin and aluminum-magnesium antacids may decrease bioavailability of atenolol.
Anticholinergic drugs may increase absorption of atenolol.

Monitor: Blood pressure, heart rate.

AZLOCILLIN (Azlin)
(Other antibiotics with similar spectrum of action: carbenicillin, mezlocillin, piperacillin, ticarcillin)

Pharmacologic Class: Anti-pseudomonas penicillin.

Mechanism of Action: Bactericidal effect due to inhibition of synthesis of cell-wall mucopeptide.

Indications:
Infections caused by susceptible organisms: *Pseudomonas aeruginosa, Klebsiella, E. coli, H. influenzae, Proteus mirabilis, Streptococcus faecalis.*
Often used in combination therapy with aminoglycoside or cephalosporin.

Pharmacokinetics:
Administered only intravenously.
50–70% excreted unchanged by kidney.
Half-life 0.8–1.3 hr, duration 4–6 hr.

Dosage:
Adult: 2–4 g every 4–6 hr; daily dose 8–18 g.
Pediatric: 75 mg/kg every 4 hr; max. 24 g daily.
Reduce dose for patients with renal failure (Cr Cl $<$ 30 ml/min).

Adverse Reactions:
Rash, fever, anaphylaxis, **diarrhea,** hepatotoxicity, nausea; superinfection; hypokalemic metabolic alkalosis; blood dyscrasia; seizure.

Contraindication: Hypersensitivity to penicillins.

Precautions: Cross-sensitivity to penicillins and cephalosporins.

Drug Interactions:
Probenecid decreases renal excretion, causing increased blood levels.
Diuretics, corticosteroids, and amphotericin B may increase the risk of hypokalemia.

Monitor: Temperature, WBC, culture and sensitivity.

BISACODYL (Dulcolax)

Pharmacologic Class: Irritant cathartic.

Mechanism of Action: Alters water and electrolyte secretion along the colon mucosa. Stimulates peristalsis.

Indication: Constipation and preparation to evacuate bowel prior to radiographic studies or surgery.

Pharmacokinetics: Direct local action on colon with minimal absorption. Effect within 15–60 min following rectal administration, 6–12 hr following oral administration.

Dosage:

	Oral	Rectal
Adult	10–15 mg hs or before breakfast	10 mg
Pediatric >6yr	5–10 mg hs or before breakfast	<2 yr 5 mg

Side Effects:
Nausea, vomiting, **abdominal cramps,** diarrhea.
Chronic use may lead to excessive loss of potassium, sodium, water.
Volume losses could result in hypotension, circulatory collapse.

Precautions:
Instruct patient to swallow whole tablet; do not chew.
Avoid in pregnancy and during lactation.
Do not use suppositories in patients with anal fissures.

Contraindications: Obstruction or acute abdomen, hypersensitivity.

Drug Interactions: Antacids may remove enteric coating on bisacodyl tablets.

Monitor: Bowel movements.

CALCIUM CARBONATE (Chooz, Titralac, Tums)
(Oral calcium salts)

Pharmacologic Class: Electrolyte supplement; nonsystemic-nonbuffer antacid; antacid.

Mechanism of Action: Nutritional supplement absorbed across GI tract. Antacid which neutralizes gastric acidity. Locally binds phosphorus to form calcium phosphate, which is eliminated in stool.

Indication:
Treatment and prevention of hypocalcemia.
Prevention of osteoporosis.
Symptomatic relief of indigestion.
Treatment and prevention of hyperphosphatemia in renal failure.

Dosage:
1–2 g of elemental calcium daily.

	% Calcium
Calcium carbonate	40
Calcium glubionate	6.5
Calcium gluconate	9
Calcium lactate	13
Dibasic calcium phosphate	23
Tricalcium phosphate	39

Side Effects:
Anorexia, nausea, vomiting, **constipation,** nephrocalcinosis, renal calculi; carbonate salts may cause abdominal gaseous distention, belching.
Hypophosphatemia possible with excessive use.

Precautions:
Avoid use with severe hyperphosphatemia (>7 mg/dl).
Chronic use may lead to milk alkali syndrome.

Contraindications: Renal calculi, hypercalcemia.

Drug Interactions:
Corticosteroids may decrease absorption of calcium salts.
Calcium salts decrease absorption of oral tetracyclines.
Calcium carbonate may decrease absorption of oral iron.

Monitor: Calcium, phosphorus; albumin, alkaline phosphatase, PTH.

CAPTOPRIL (Capoten)
(Other similar agents: enalapril, lisinopril)

Pharmacologic Class: Angiotension converting enzyme inhibitors.

Mechanism of Action: Inhibition of conversion of angiotensin I to angiotensin II, a potent vasoconstrictor which also stimulates the release of aldosterone.

Indications:
Hypertension.
Congestive heart failure.

Route of Excretion: 75% absorbed from GI tract, peak levels 0.5–1.5 hr, duration 6–12 hr; 50% excreted unchanged by kidneys.

Dosage:
HT: initial dose 25 mg bid–tid, titrate dose.
CHF: initial dose 6.25–25 mg tid, titrate dose.
Maximum dose 150 mg tid

Precautions:
Dosage reduction in patients with renal insufficiency.
Greater risk of neutropenia in patients with renal insufficiency and collagen vascular disease, especially at higher doses.
Use with caution during surgery/anesthesia and in patients with aortic valvular stenosis.
Acute renal insufficiency, especially in patients with bilateral renal artery stenosis and volume depletion.
Proteinuria and nephrotic syndrome (membranous glomerulopathy) more likely in patients with prior renal disease.
Hyperkalemia may occur, especially in patients with renal insufficiency, diabetes mellitus, and potassium-sparing drugs.

Contraindications: Hypersensitivity.

Adverse reactions: Proteinuria, nephrotic syndrome, membranous glomerulopathy, acute renal insufficiency; rash; anorexia, **dysgeusia,** dry mouth; blood dyscrasias (neutropenia); **hypotension,** tachycardia.

Drug Interactions:
Additive hypotension with other antihypertensives.
Concomitant diuretics may cause precipitous drop in blood pressure with initial dose and may increase risk of acute renal insufficiency in patients with bilateral renal artery stenosis.
Potassium-sparing diuretics, potassium supplements, and salt substitutes may increase risk of hyperkalemia.
Nonsteroidal anti-inflammatory agents may blunt antihypertensive effect of captopril.

Monitor: Blood pressure, heart rate, proteinuria, BUN, creatinine, potassium, WBC with differential.

CARBAMAZEPINE (Tegretol)

Pharmacologic Class: Anticonvulsant.

Mechanism of Action: Decreases synaptic responses and blocks post-tetanic potentiation. Stimulates release of ADH.

Indications:
Refractory seizure disorders: partial complex, generalized tonic-clonic, or mixed seizure pattern.
Trigeminal neuralgia.
Partial central diabetes insipidus.

Route of Excretion: Extensive hepatic metabolism.

Dosage:
Adult: Initial 200 mg bid, titrate to maximum 1200 mg daily in 3–4 divided doses.
Pediatric (6–12 yr): 20–30 mg/kg/day in 2–4 divided doses. Therapeutic serum concentrations 4–12 mcg/ml.

Adverse Reactions: Dizziness, drowsiness, ataxia, headache, confusion, hallucinations; diplopia, blurred vision; nausea, vomiting, hepatotoxicity; blood dyscrasias (leukopenia, aplastic anemia, thrombocytopenia); urinary frequency, retention; azotemia, proteinuria; rash, fever, pulmonary hypersensitivity.

Contraindications:
Hypersensitivity to carbamazepine or tricyclic antidepressants.
History of bone marrow depression.
Concomitant use of MAO inhibitors.

Precautions:
Use with caution in patients with cardiac, hepatic, or renal disease; prostatic hypertrophy; or glaucoma.
Caution for patients driving or operating heavy machinery due to drowsiness and blurred vision.

Drug Interactions:
Increase serum levels of carbamazepine by troleandomycin, erythromycin, cimetidine, isoniazid, or propoxyphene.
Carbamazepine may also increase risk of isoniazid-induced hepatotoxicity.
Decreased carbamazepine serum levels by phenobarbital, phenytoin, or primidone.
Carbamazepine may enhance metabolism of warfarin, oral contraceptives, phenytoin, ethosuximide, valproic acid, doxycycline, or theophylline.
Carbamazepine may increase therapeutic or toxic effect of lithium therapy.

Monitor: Serum carbamazepine concentrations (normal 4–12 mcg/ml) LFTs, CBC, BUN, creatinine, proteinuria, baseline and periodic eye exams.

CEFAZOLIN (Ancef, Kefzol)
(Other agents with similar spectrum: cefaclor, cefadroxil, cephalexin, cephalothin, cephapirin, cephradine)

Pharmacologic Class: First-generation cephalosporins.

Mechanism of Action: Inhibit formation of bacterial cell wall, causing lysis of cell.

Indications: Infections caused by susceptible organisms: *Staphylococci* (except methicillin-resistant staph), *Streptococcus pneumoniae*, beta-hemolytic streptococci, *E. coli, H. influenzae, Klebsiella, Proteus mirabilis*.

Dosage:
Adult: 0.25–2.0 g IV/IM q 6–8 hr.
Pediatric (>1 mo): 25–100 mg/kg in 3–4 divided doses.
Reduce dose in patients with impaired renal function.

Adverse Reactions: Rash, urticaria, fever, anaphylaxis; **nausea, vomiting, diarrhea,** pseudomembranous colitis; blood dyscrasias, Coomb's positivity; superinfection; seizures (at excessive doses); phlebitis; pain at IM site; transient liver enzyme abnormalities.

Precautions:
Cross-allergenicity with penicillins.
Does not penetrate into CSF.
Do not use for patients with methicillin-resistant staphylococci.

Contraindication: Hypersensitivity to cephalosporins or severe penicillin allergy.

Drug Interactions:
Probenecid decreases renal excretion and increases plasma levels.
May potentiate nephrotoxicity by other drugs.

Monitor: Temperature, WBC, culture and sensitivity.

CEFOXITIN (Mefoxin)
(Other agents with similar spectrum: cefamandole, cefuroxime, cefaclor, ceforanide, cefonicid)

Pharmacologic Class: Second-generation cephalosporin.

Mechanism of Action: Inhibit formation of bacterial cell wall, causing lysis of cell.

Indications: Infections caused by susceptible organisms: *Staphylococci, Streptococcus pneumoniae*, beta-hemolytic streptococci, *E. coli, H. influenzae, Klebsiella, Proteus, Providencia, Clostridium, B. fragilis, Serratia marcescens, Peptococcus, Peptostreptococcus.*

Pharmacokinetics: Primarily excreted unchanged by kidneys, $t^{1/2}$ 0.5–1.0 hr, peak serum after 1 g IV 85–100 mcg/ml, duration 4–6 hr.

Dosage:
Adult: 1–2 g IV/IM q 6–8 hr.
Pediatric (>3 mo): 80–160 mg/kg/d in 4–6 divided doses.
Reduce dose in patients with impaired renal function.

Adverse Reactions: Rash, urticaria, fever, anaphylaxis; **nausea,** vomiting, **diarrhea,** pseudomembranous colitis; blood dyscrasias, Coomb's positivity; superinfection; seizures (at excessive doses); phlebitis; pain at IM sites; transient liver enzyme abnormalities.

Precautions:
Cross-allergenicity with penicillins.
Does not penetrate into CSF.
Do not use for patients with methicillin-resistant staphylococci.

Contraindications: Hypersensitivity to cephalosporins or severe penicillin allergy.

Drug Interactions:
Probenecid decreases renal excretion and increases plasma levels.
May potentiate nephrotoxicity by other drugs.

Monitor: Temperature, WBC, culture and sensitivity.

CEFTRIAXONE (Rocephin)
(Other agents with similar spectrum: cefoperazone, cefotetan, ceforanide, cefotaxime, ceftazidime, ceftizoxime, moxalactam)

Pharmacologic Class: Third-generation cephalosporin.

Mechanism of Action: Inhibit formation of bacterial cell wall, causing lysis of cell.

Indications:
Infections caused by susceptible organisms: *Staphylococci, Streptococcus pneumoniae*, beta-hemolytic *Streptococci, E. coli, H. influenzae, Klebsiella, Proteus, Enterobacter, Pseudomonas aeruginosa, Serratia, Neisseria, Providentia pseudomonas, B. fragilis.*

Pharmacokinetics: $1/3$–$2/3$ of dose excreted unchanged by kidneys, $t^{1}/_{2}$ 6.0–8.5 hr; peak serum after 1 g IV 150 mcg/ml, duration 12–24 hr.

Dosage:
Adult: 1–2 g IV/IM q 12–24 hr.
Pediatric: 50–100 mg/kg/d in 2 divided doses.
No dosage adjustment is needed for renal or hepatic impairment.

Adverse Reactions: **Rash**, urticaria, fever, anaphylaxis; nausea, vomiting, **diarrhea,** pseudomembranous colitis; blood dyscrasias, Coomb's positivity, altered prothrombin times; superinfection; seizures (at excessive doses); phlebitis; pain at IM sites; transient liver enzyme abnormalities.

Precautions:
Cross-allergenicity with penicillins.
Do not use for patients with methicillin-resistant staphylococci.

Contraindications: Hypersensitivity to cephalosporins or severe penicillin allergy.

Drug Interactions: May potentiate nephrotoxicity by other drugs.

Monitor: Temperature, WBC, culture and sensitivity.

CHLORPROMAZINE (Promapar, Thorazine)

Pharmacologic Class: Phenothiazine antipsychotic.

Mechanism of Action: Blocks α-adrenoceptors and dopamine-2 receptors in the brain.

Indications:
Treatment of psychotic disorders.
Control of nausea, vomiting, and intractable hiccoughs.

Pharmacokinetics:
Variable oral absorption, improved with oral liquid formations, more erratic with controlled release capsules, good IM absorption.
Extensively metabolized by the liver.
Half-life 30 hr.

Dosage:
Adult—psychosis
  Oral: 30–1000 mg in 1–4 divided doses.
  IM: 25 mg, repeat 1–4 hr prn.
Adult—nausea and vomiting
  Oral: 10–25 mg q 4–6 hr prn.
  Rectal: 50–100 mg q 6–8 hr prn.
  IM: 25–50 mg q 3–4 hr prn.
Adult—intractable hiccoughs
  Oral: 25–50 mg tid–qid.
  IM: (if no response to po): same dose.
  IV: 25–50 mg in 500–1000 ml PSS.
Pediatric >6 mo
  Oral: 0.5 mg/kg q 4–6 hr.
  IM: 0.5 mg q 6–8 hr.
  Rectal: 1 mg/kg q 6–8 hr.

Adverse Reactions: Sedation, depression, **extrapyramidal reactions,** seizures, tardive dyskinesia; **orthostatic hypotension,** tachycardia; CHF, arrhythmias; **urticaria,** rash, **photosensitivity, skin pigmentation;** infertility, impotence, gynecomastia, amenorrhea, galactorrhea; **dry mouth, weight gain,** constipation, cholestatic jaundice; urinary retention; blood dyscrasias (leukopenia); malignant hyperthermia.

Precautions:
Use cautiously in elderly and patients with prostatic hypertrophy, seizure disorder, glaucoma.
Tardive dyskinesias are most likely to develop in patients treated with high cumulative doses for long duration.
Drowsiness is greatest during first 2 weeks of therapy. Caution patients concerning driving and operating hazardous machinery.
Discontinue phenothiazines for 48 hr prior and 24 hr after myelography.

Drug Interactions:
Barbiturates, smoking may increase metabolism of chlorpromazine. Propranolol may decrease metabolism of chlorpromazine.

Decreased absorption of phenothiazines by antacids, anticholinergics.

Phenothiazines may inhibit metabolism of tricyclics, phenytoin, propranolol.

Phenothiazines may inhibit effect of levodopa, guanethidine, amphetamine, chlorphentiramine, or phenmetrazine.

Amphetamines, anticholinergics may inhibit antipsychotic effect of phenothiazine.

Lithium may alter response to chlorpromazine and vice versa. Potential increased neurotoxicity.

Antipsychotics may increase effect of antihypertensives, CNS depressants, and anticholinergics.

Monitor: Symptomatic response, WBC (wk 4–10), LFTs (wk 2–4), extrapyramidal reactions.

CIMETIDINE (Tagamet)

Pharmacologic Class: H_2-receptor antagonist.

Mechanism of Action: Inhibits histamine-stimulated gastric acid secretion.

Indications:
Prophylaxis and treatment of duodenal ulcer.
Treatment of active benign gastric ulcers.
Zollinger-Ellison syndrome.
Systemic mastocytosis.
Also used in prevention of stress ulcers, acute upper GI bleeding, GE reflux.

Route of Excretion: Primarily excreted unchanged by kidney, 30% metabolized in the liver.

Dosage:
Treatment of active ulcer
  Oral: 300 mg qid, 400 mg bid, 800 mg hs.
  IV/IM: 300 mg q 6 hr.
Prophylaxis of duodenal ulcer: 400 mg hs.
Zollinger Ellison: 300–600 mg po/IV/IM q 6 hr.
Reduce dose in elderly and patients with renal insufficiency.

Adverse Reactions: Sedation, dizziness, headache; rash; **diarrhea,** hepatitis; gynecomastia, impotence; blood dyscrasias.

Precautions:
Rapid IV administration has rarely been associated with hypotension and arrhythmias.
Cimetidine inhibits tubular secretion of creatinine and may raise serum creatinine without changing GFR.

Contraindications: Hypersensitivity.

Drug Interactions:
Cimetidine may decrease metabolism of warfarin, cyclosporine, theophylline, phenytoin, carbamazepine, lidocaine, quinidine, caffeine, ethanol, tricyclic antidepressants, meperidine, fentanyl, some beta blockers (metoprolol, propranolol), some benzodiazepines (alprazolam, chlordiazepoxide, diazepam, flurazepam, and temazepam).
Cimetidine may decrease the renal clearance of procainamide.
Cimetidine may decrease the absorption of ketoconazole.
Antacids, metaclopramide may decrease the absorption of cimetidine.

CLINDAMYCIN (Cleocin)
(Other agents with similar spectrum of action: lincomycin)

Pharmacologic Class: Lincosamide antibiotic.

Mechanism of Action: Inhibits protein synthesis by binding to the 50S subunit of bacterial ribosomes.

Indications:
Infections caused by susceptible organisms: *Staphylococcus, Streptococcus pneumoniae, Cornyebacterium diptheriae, Nocardia*, and anaerobes, including *Bacteroides* and *Clostridium*, especially *B. fragilis* (non-CNS).
Used topically for severe acne vulgaris.

Pharmacokinetics:
Mostly metabolized by the liver, $t^{1/2}$ 2–3 hr, peak after 300 mg: 4 (oral), 5 (IM), 15 (IV) mcg/ml; duration 6–8 hr.
Does not penetrate into CSF.
Minimal absorption of topical solution.

Dosage:

	Adult	Pediatric
Oral	150–450 mg q 6 hr	8–25 mg/kg/day in 3–4 divided doses.
IM/IV over 30–60 min.	600–2700 mg in 2–4 divided doses	15–40 mg/kg/day in 3–4 divided doses

May require dosage reduction with severe hepatic dysfunction.
Topical (1% sol), apply bid.

Adverse Reactions: Nausea, vomiting, **diarrhea,** pseudomembranous colitis; rash; hypotension and arrhythmias with IV bolus; phlebitis (IV), sterile abscess (IM).

Precautions:
Should not be used against Gram-positive cocci if penicillin or erythromycin can be used.
May cause pseudomembranous colitis (greater risk with oral therapy).
Use cautiously in patients with severe liver disease.

Contraindications: Hypersensitivity.

Drug Interactions: Clindamycin may enhance neuromuscular blockade in patients treated with neuromuscular blocking agents.
Kaolin may decrease GI absorption of clindamycin.

Monitor: Temperature, WBC, culture and sensitivity, bowel movements.

CLONIDINE (Catapres)

Pharmacologic Class: α_1- and α_2-adrenoceptor agonist.

Mechanism of Action: Clonidine is a central alpha-adrenergic stimulant with results in decrease in blood pressure and heart rate.

Indications:
Hypertension.
Migraine headache prophylaxis.
Dysmenorrhea.
Diabetic diarrhea.
Withdrawal of alcohol, benzodiazepines, methadone, and opiates.

Pharmacodynamics:

	Onset	Peak	Duration
oral	30–60 min	2–5 hr	8 hr
topical	2–3 d	unknown	7 d

Route of Excretion: 40–60% of absorbed dose is excreted unchanged in the urine, approximately 50% metabolized by liver.

Dosage: 0.1–2.4 mg/day in 2–3 divided doses. Initial dose 0.1 mg bid.

Adverse Reactions: Drowsiness, sedation, depression, headache; **dry mouth,** constipation; fluid retention, weight gain; impotence; rash; anorexia, vivid dreams, stimulation of CNS.

Precautions:
Withdraw gradually to prevent rebound hypertension.
Use with caution with patients with depression; renal, cardiac, or cerebrovascular disease.

Contraindications: Hypersensitivity.

Drug Interactions:
Clonidine withdraw may result in rebound hypertension in patients treated with beta blockers.
Tricyclic antidepressants may block the antihypertensive effect of clonidine.
Enhanced CNS depression with alcohol, barbiturates, and narcotics.

Monitor: Blood pressure, heart rate.

CYCLOPHOSPHAMIDE (Cytoxan, Neosar)

Pharmacologic Class: Alkylating agent, antineoplastic, immunosuppressant.

Mechanism of Action: Inhibition of DNA/RNA synthesis of protein by an active metabolite, phosphoramide mustard by alkylation. At low doses, immunosuppression by inhibition of B lymphocytes.

Indications: Used alone or in combination as an antineoplastic for malignant lymphomas, leukemias, multiple myeloma, breast and ovarian cancer, mycosis fungoides, advanced neuroblastoma, retinoblastoma; immunosuppressive agent, often in combination with corticosteroids for Wegener's granulomatosis, systemic lupus erythematosus, nephrotic syndrome, rheumatoid arthritis, and other vasculidites.

Route of Excretion: Metabolized to active drug by the liver; 30 % excreted renally as unchanged drug.

Dosage:
Reduction: 40–50 mg/kg in divided doses over 2–5 days, oral 1–5 mg/kg/day.
Maintenance: IV, 10–15 mg/kg q 7–10 days or 3–5 mg/kg twice weekly; oral, 1–5 mg/kg/day.
Reduced doses for patients with severe renal or hepatic dysfunction, tumor infiltration of bone marrow, or previous cytoxic or radiation therapy which may have decreased bone marrow reserve.

Adverse Reactions: Alopecia, impaired skin healing; **anorexia, nausea, vomiting, diarrhea, stomatitis,** cardiotoxicity, pulmonary fibrosis, **leukopenia** (7–21 days post-therapy), thrombocytopenia, anemia, secondary neoplasma, **hemorrhagic cystitis, hematuria,** SIADH($>$50 mg/kg IV), hyperuricemia, hyperpigmentation.

Precautions:
Increased fluid intake and frequent voiding may prevent hemorrhagic cystitis.
Use cautiously in patients with infections, bone marrow suppression, or impaired hepatic or renal function.
May be carcinogenic with long-term use.

Contraindications: Hypersensitivity, avoid during pregnancy and lactation.

Drug Interactions:
Phenobarbital, allopurinol, and thiazides may increase the risk of leukopenia.
Chloramphemicol may reduce the effect of cyclophosphamide.
Cyclophosphamide may inhibit metabolism and enhance effect of succinylcholine.

Monitor: CBC, uric acid, urine output, urinalysis.

CYCLOSPORINE (Sandimmune)

Pharmacologic Class: Immunosuppressant.

Mechanism of Action: Inhibition of interleukin-2, causing suppression of T lymphocytes (T helper > T suppressor), which mediate rejection reaction.

Indication: Prophylaxis of rejection in organ transplantation.

Pharmacokinetics:
Bioavailability approximately 37% of oral dose; extensively metabolized by liver by cytochrome P-450 to probably inactive metabolites and excreted in bile, 6% excreted renally as unchanged drug; widely distributed, approximately 90% bound to proteins (lipoproteins); half-life 10–27 hours.
Therapeutic concentrations: 100–200 ng/ml (HPLC, whole blood), 250–800 ng/ml (RIA, whole blood), 50–300 (RIA, plasma).

Dosage:
Oral: 5–15 mg/kg/d.
IV: 1/3 oral dose, 2–5 mg/kg/d.
Adjust to drug concentrations.

Administration:
Dilute oral suspension in milk, chocolate milk, or orange juice to improve palatability of olive oil suspension. Do not use Styrofoam cups.
Administer IV cyclosporine as slow intravenous infusion over 2–6 hours in 5% dextrose or 0.9% NaCl.

Adverse Reactions: Nephrotoxicity, hyperkalemia, hyperuricemia, hypomagnesemia; **hirsutism, gingival hyperplasia; tremor,** seizures; **hypertension;** nausea, vomiting, diarrhea, hepatotoxicity; infections; lymphoma; hypersensitivity, including anaphylaxis.

Precautions:
Frequent adverse reactions; monitor patient carefully.
Therapeutic concentration varies with method of cyclosporine assay.

Contraindications: Hypersensitivity to cyclosporine or polyoxyethylated castor oil (IV vehicle).

Drug Interactions:
Increased cyclosporine concentrations due to inhibition of cytochrome P-450 by ketoconazole, erythromycin, cimetidine, diltiazem.
Decreased cyclosporine concentrations due to enhanced metabolism by phenytoin, phenobarbital, rifampin.
Increased risk of nephrotoxicity with aminoglycosides, amphotericin B, melphalan, sulfamethoxazole/trimethoprim.

Monitor: Cyclosporine concentrations; BUN, creatinine, potassium; blood pressure; LFTs.

DEXAMETHASONE (Decadron, Hexadrol)

Pharmacologic Class: Glucocorticoid—long acting.

Mechanism of Action: Anti-inflammatory action and immunosuppressant effect due to a variety of effects such as inhibition of protein synthesis, inhibition of prostaglandin synthesis, impaired cell-mediated immunity by reduction in T lymphocytes, decreased neutrophil migration, decreased capillary permeability, vasoconstriction.

Indications:
Used for autoimmune, allergic, and inflammatory disorders, malignancies.
Suppression test for Cushing's syndrome.
Management of cerebral edema.
Septic shock.
Antiemetic.
Diagnosis of depression.

Route of Excretion: Hepatically metabolized with plasma half-life 110–120 min; biologic half-life 36–54 hr.

Dosage: 0.75 mg dexamethasone adult equivalent to 25 mg cortisone; child equivalent to 5 mg prednisone.

	Adult	Pediatric
Oral	0.5–9.0 mg in 2–4 divided doses	2.5–10 mg/m^2/d in 3–4 divided doses
IM/IV	0.5–24 mg/day in 2–4 divided doses	1–5 mg/m^2/d in 3–4 divided doses

Side Effects: Adrenal suppression, stunted growth in children, depression, euphoria, insomnia, psychoses, moon facies, buffalo hump, **hirsutism, impaired wound healing, petechiae, ecchymoses,** hyperpigmentation, glaucoma, cataracts; weight gain, nausea, vomiting, azotemia; peptic ulceration, pancreatitis; **hyperglycemia,** amenorrhea; thromboembolism; myopathy, osteoporosis, infections.

Precautions:
Chronic use leads to adrenal suppression; patients will require supplemental doses during stress; do not discontinue abruptly.
May mask signs of infections, may reactivate latent TB; may exacerbate fungal infections.
Monitor glucose carefully in patients with diabetes mellitus or latent DM.
Avoid use in patients with psychosis, osteoporosis, glaucoma, or ulcer disease if possible.

Contraindications: Systemic fungal infections, administration of live virus vaccines.

Drug Interactions:
Phenobarbital, phenytoin, and rifampin increase metabolism and

may decrease effect of dexamethasone.
Estrogens (oral contraceptives), isoniazid, and troleandomycin may inhibit steroid metabolism.
Increased requirement for insulin and oral hypoglycemics in diabetics.
Inhibition of coumadin response by steroids.
Enchanced metabolism of isoniazid and reduced effect of INH.

Monitor: WBC with differential.

DIAZEPAM (Valium)

Pharmacologic Class: Benzodiazepine.

Mechanism of Action: CNS depressant by unknown mechanism. Depress limbic systems and reticular formation, brainstem, and spinal cord. Skeletal muscle relaxation. Potentiate GABA.

Indications:
Sedative/hypnotic.
Anticonvulsant.
Skeletal muscle relaxant.
Symptoms of alcohol withdrawal.

Route of Excretion: Metabolized by the liver to desmethyldiazepam (active) and other metabolites; half-life 20–50 hr.

Dosage:

Adult	Pediatric
Oral: 2–10 mg bid–qid	1–2.5 mg tid–qid
IV/IM: 2–20 mg	0.2–1.0 mg

Precautions:
Prolonged administration may lead to dependence. Use cautiously in depressed or suicidal patients.
Use cautiously in patients with hepatic or renal dysfunction, children, elderly or debilitated patients.

Contraindicated: Hypersensitivity, acute narrow-angle glaucoma.

Side Effects: Drowsiness, lethargy, dizziness, ataxia, depression, paradoxical excitation; blurred vision; dry mouth, nausea, vomiting, diarrhea, constipation, respiratory depression, hypotension, arrhythmias, rash, phlebitis (IV), pain, erythema (IM).

Drug Interactions:
Cimetidine, isoniazid, disulfiram, oral contraceptives and valproic acid may impair diazepam's metabolism.
Rifampin and barbiturates may increase metabolism of diazepam.
Additive CNS depression with alcohol, antihistamines, antidepressants, barbiturates, and narcotics.
Effectiveness of levodopa may be decreased by benzodiazepines.

Monitor: CNS effect.

DIGOXIN (Lanoxin)

Pharmacologic Class: Cardiac glycoside, antiarrhythmic.

Mechanism of Action: Enhanced myocardial contractility (positive inotropic effect) through increased intracellular calcium and release of calcium from binding sites on sarcoplasmic reticulum. Depress SA node with slowed conduction to AV node (negative chronotropic effect).

Indications:
Congestive heart failure.
Atrial arrhythmias (atrial fibrillation, flutter, and paroxysmal atrial tachycardia).

Pharmacokinetics: Absorption: Tablets/elixir, 55–85%; liquid capsules, 90–100%; renally eliminated t 1/2 30–44 hr; therapeutic concentration equals 0.5–2.0 ng/ml.

Pharmacodynamics:

	Onset	Peak	Duration
oral	30–120 min	2–6 hr	2–4 days
IV	5–30 min	1–5 hr	2–4 days

Dosage:
Adult: loading, 8–15 mcg/kg (50% initial, 25% q 4–8 hr × 2 doses); maintenance, 0.125–0.5 mg/day.
Pediatric: loading, oral: >10 yr, 10–15 mcg/kg; 5–10 yr, 20–35 mcg/kg; 2–5 yr, 30–40 mcg/kg; 1–24 mo, 35–60 mcg/kg; 0–1 mo, 25–35 mcg/kg, premature, 20–30 mcg/kg. IV, give 10% of oral/next-day dose. Maintenance, 25–30% of loading dose; premature infant, 20–30% of loading dose.
Reduced doses with renal insufficiency and myxedema.
Increased doses with thyrotoxic patients.

Side Effects: **Anorexia, nausea, vomiting,** diarrhea; fatigue; rash; blurred or yellow vision; gynecomastia, **bradycardia**, thrombocytopenia.

Precautions:
Hypokalemia, hypercalemia, and hypomagnesemia, increases risk of digoxin toxicity.
Premature infants and patients with severe pulmonary disease, myocardial infarction, or severe heart failure may demonstrate increased sensitivity to digoxin.
Do not administer IV calcium to digitalized patients.

Contraindications: Hypersensitivity, digitalis intoxication, uncontrolled ventricular tachycardia or fibrillation, AV block.

Drug Interactions:
Quinidine, verapamil, spironolactone, or nifedipine increases digoxin

levels.

Potassium-wasting duiretics, carbenicillin/ticarcillin, amphotericin B, aminoglycosides, and corticosteroids may cause hypokalemia and increase risk of digoxin toxicity.

Additive bradycardia with beta blockers and succinylcholine.

Antacids, cholestyramine, colestipol, oral aminoglycosides, sulfasalazine, metoclopramide, and kaolin-pectin may decrease digoxin absorption.

Propantheline may increase the absorption of digoxin.

Monitor: Heart rate, serum concentrations, ECG, potassium, creatinine (pretreatment).

DILTIAZEM (Cardizem)

Pharmacologic Class: Calcium channel antagonist, coronary vasodilator.

Mechanism of Action: Coronary vasodilation due to inhibition of calcium entry into vascular and myocardial smooth muscles.

Indications:
Angina pectoris.
Hypertension.

Route of Excretion: Rapidly metabolized by the liver to active metabolite. Duration 6–8 hr.

Dosage: 120–240 mg in 3–4 divided doses.

Adverse Reactions: Edema, rash, headache, dizziness, **fatigue,** arrhythmias, hypotention; **nausea,** constipation, hepatitis.

Precautions: Use with caution in patients with severe liver disease.

Contraindications: Sick sinus syndrome, second- and third-degree heart block.

Drug Interactions:
Increased risk of bradycardia with beta blockers or digoxin.
Diltiazem may decrease metabolism and result in increased cyclosporine concentrations.
Cimetidine and propranolol may decrease metabolism of diltiazem and enhance its effect.
Phenobarbital and phenytoin may increase metabolism of diltiazem and decrease its effect.

Monitor: Blood pressure, heart rate.

DIPHENHYDRAMINE (Benadryl, Benylin)

Pharmacologic Class: Ethanolamine antihistamines.

Mechanism of Action: Competitive antagonism of histamine at H_1 receptor.

Indications:
Symptomatic relief of allergic reactions.
Prophylaxis of motion sickness.
Cough suppressant.
Parkinsonism.
Sedative.

Route of Excretion: Metabolized by the liver.

Dosage:

	Oral	IV/IM
Adult	25–50 mg tid–qid	10–50 mg/dose ($\not\gt$ 400 mg/day)
Pediatric (>10 kg)	12.5–25 mg tid–qid	5 mg/kg/day in 3–4 divided doses ($\not\gt$ 300 mg/day)

Side Effects: Sedation, drowsiness, dizziness, paradoxical excitation; **dry mouth,** anorexia, weight gain; blurred vision; urinary retention; hypotension, palpitations; thickening of bronchial secretions, respiratory depression.

Precautions:
Due to anticholinergic effect, use with caution in elderly and in patients with prostatic hypertrophy, seizure disorder, narrow-angle glaucoma.
Warn patients about sedative effect when driving or operating hazardous machinery.

Contraindications: Acute asthmatic attack.

Drug Interactions:
Additive CNS depression with alcohol, narcotics, barbiturates, antidepressants, sedative/hypnotics.
Additive anticholinergic properties with MAO inhibitors.
Epinephrine effect may be enhanced by diphenhydramine.

DIPHENOXYLATE with ATROPINE (Lomotil)

Pharmacologic Class: Antidiarrheal narcotic.

Mechanism of Action: Decreased motility of colon by this meperidine congener without analgesic properties.

Indications: Adjunctive treatment of diarrhea.

Route of Excretion: Metabolized by the liver to active metabolite.

Dosage:
Equivalent antidiarrheal activity to 30–45 mg codeine.
Adult: 5–20 mg/day in 1–4 divided doses.
Pediatric: (8–12 yr) 10 mg in 5 divided doses; (5–8 yr) 8 mg in 4 divided doses; (2–5 yr) 6 mg in 3 divided doses.

Adverse Reactions: Dizziness, drowsiness; anorexia, nausea, vomiting, dry mouth, **constipation,** ileus; flushing; blurred vision; tachycardia; urinary retention.

Precautions: Atropine has been added in subtherapeutic doses (0.025 mg/2.5 mg diphenoxylate) to discourage abuse.

Contraindications: Diarrhea associated with pseudomembranous colitis.
Severe liver disease.
Hypersensitivity.
Children <2 yr.

Drug Interactions:
Additive CNS depression with alcohol, barbiturates, antihistamines, narcotics, sedatives/hypnotics.
Concurrent use with MAO inhibitors may precipitate hypertensive crisis.

DOCUSATE (Sodium: Colace, Doxinate; Calcium: Surfak; Potassium-Dialose)

Pharmacologic Class: Stool softener.

Mechanism of Action: Detergent properties promote incorporation of water into feces.

Indications: Prevention of constipation.

Route of Excretion: Poorly absorbed, absorbed drug eliminated in bile.

Dosage:
Adult: 50–300 mg/day.
Pediatric: (2–12 yr) 50–150 mg/day; (<2 yr) 25 mg/day.
Onset of action 24–72 hours.

Side Effects: Diarrhea, abdominal cramps.

Contraindications: Acute abdomen.

Drug Interactions: Docusate may increase absorption of danthron and mineral oil and increase risk of hepatotoxicity.

DOPAMINE (Intropin)

Pharmacologic Class: Inotropic agent, vasopressor.

Mechanism of Action: An endogenous catecholamine and precursor of norepinephrine with dose-related effects. It produces vasodilation by activating dopaminergic receptor at low doses (0.5–2 mcg/kg/min). Intermediate doses (2–10 mcg/kg/min) stimulate beta-adrenergic and dopaminergic receptors, thus increasing cardiac output and renal blood flow. At higher doses (>10 mcg/kg/min), alpha-adrenergic activity predominates, causing vasoconstriction.

Indications: For treatment of shock and severe congestive heart failure to increase cardiac output, blood pressure, and glomerular filtration rate.

Pharmacodynamics: IV: onset 2–5 minutes, duration <10 minutes.

Route of Excretion: Metabolized by liver, small amount of drug is excreted renally unchanged.

Dosage:
Titrate dose by response.
Initiate therapy at 1–5 mcg/kg/min, maximum 50 mcg/kg/min.

Adverse Reactions: Headache; **tachycardia, hypotension,** hypertension, palpitations, angina, vasoconstriction; dyspnea; nausea, vomiting, piloerection, phlebitis, necrosis.

Precautions:
Use cautiously in patients with occlusive vascular disease.
Infuse into large vein to decrease risk of phlebitis and extravasation.
Use as adjunctive therapy in patients who have been appropriately replaced with fluid volume.

Contraindications: Pheochromocytoma, tachyarrhythmias.

Drug Interactions:
Tricyclics, MAO inhibitors, and ergot alkaloids may potentiate pressor response of dopamine.
Cycloproprane and halogenated anesthetics may increase risk of arrhythmias and pressor response.
Beta blockers may antagonize dopamine's effect.
IV phenytoin concomitantly with dopamine may cause hypotension, bradycardia, and seizures.

Monitor: Blood pressure, urine output, cardiac output, heart rate, ECG.

DOXORUBICIN (Adriamycin)

Pharmacologic Class: Antineoplastic anthracycline antibiotic.

Mechanism of Action: Inhibition of DNA and RNA synthesis by binding to DNA.

Indications: Used alone or in combination as an antineoplastic for leukemias; lymphomas; Wilm's tumor; neuroblastoma; carcinoma of breast, ovary, bladder, lung (small cell), thyroid.

Route of Excretion: Metabolized by the liver and primarily excreted in bile.

Dosage:
Intravenous: 60–75 mg/m^2 q 21 days; 30 mg/m^2/d × 3 days q 4 wk. Do not exceed 550 mg/m^2 cumulative dose.
Reduced dose with liver impairment.

Adverse Reactions: Alopecia; **cardiomyopathy**; bone marrow suppression (**leukopenia**, anemia, thrombocytopenia); **phlebitis**; anorexia, **nausea, vomiting**, diarrhea, **stomatitis, esophagitis**; hyperuricemia; urine discoloration (red); fever, urticaria, anaphylaxis.

Precautions:
Use cautiously in patients with infections, bone marrow suppression, or impaired cardiac or hepatic function.
Increased risk of cardiotoxicity at cumulative doses >400 mg/m^2 in patients who received mediastinal radiotherapy.

Contraindications: Hypersensitivity.

Drug Interactions:
Doxorubicin may increase radiation toxicity at skin, myocardium, bone marrow, and mucosa.
Doxorubicin may increase hemorrhagic cystitis and cardiac toxicity from cyclophosphamide.
Doxorubicin may increase hepatic toxicity from 6-mercaptopurine.

Monitor: CBC, mucosa, cardiac function, cumulative dose, injection site.

ERYTHROMYCIN (Base: E-Mycin, Ery-Tab, Eryc; E. estolate: Ilosone; E. Stearate: Erypar, Ethril, Wyamycin S; E. ethylsuccinate-EES: Pediamycin, EryPed, E-MycinE, Wyamycin E)

Pharmacologic Class: Macrolide antibiotic.

Mechanism of Action: Inhibits protein synthesis by binding to the 50S subunit of bacterial ribosomes.

Indications: Infections caused by susceptible organisms: *Staphylococcus aureus, Streptococcus pneumoniae, Streptococcus pyogenes, Streptococcus viridans,* group A beta-hemolytic streptococci, *Clostridium, Corynebacterium diphtheriae, Neisseria gonorrhoeae, Hemophilus influenzae, Legionella pneumophilia, Mycoplasma pneumoniae, Listeria, Chlamydia, Treponema pallidum.* Often an alternative for penicillin allergic patients.

Route of Excretion: Metabolized by the liver, excreted primarily in the bile. Half-life 1.4–2.0 hr.

Dosage:

	Adult	Pediatric
IV	1–4 gm/d in 4 divided doses or as continuous infusion	15–20 mg/kg/d in 4 divided doses or in continuous infusion
po	(base, estolate, stearate) 250–500 mg q 6–8 hr (ethylsuccinate) 400–800 mg q 6–8 hr	30–100 mg/kg/d in 4 divided doses

Adverse Reactions: Nausea, vomiting, abdominal pain, diarrhea, cholestatic hepatitis (more common with estolate salt); reversible ototoxicity; psychiatric effects; rash, allergic reactions; phlebitis at IV site.

Precautions:
Avoid estolate salt during pregnancy.
Use cautiously in patients with impaired hepatic function.
Superinfections, including Pseudomembranous colitis, may occur.

Contraindications:
Hypersensitivity.
The estolate salt should be avoided in patients with liver dysfunction.

Drug Interactions:
Erythromycin inhibits the metabolism of theophylline, warfarin, and carbamazepine, therefore decreased doses may be needed.
Erythromycin may increase the bioavailability of digoxin in some patients; a dose reduction may be needed.

Monitor: WBC, temperature, culture and sensitivity, liver function tests.

FERROUS SALTS (F. sulfate—Mol Iron, Fer-In-Sol, Feosol; F. gluconate—Fergon)

Pharmacologic Class: Iron preparation, antianemic.

Mechanism of Action: Iron is absorbed from duodenum and upper jejuneum. It is incorporated into hemoglobin and myoglobin.

Indication: Prevention and treatment of iron-deficiency anemias.

Route of Excretion: 5–30% of iron is absorbed, remainder is eliminated in stool.

Dosage:
Elemental iron content of salts: f. gluconate, 11.6%; f. sulfate, 20%; f. fumarate, 33%.
RDA (elemental iron): adult males, 10 mg; females, 18 mg; pregnancy and lactation, 30–60 mg; children, 10–15 mg.
Replacement dose (elemental iron): 6 mg/kg/day.

	Adult	**Pediatric**
Prophylactic	300–325 mg iron salt/d	5–8 mg iron salt kg/day
Therapeutic	300–650 mg iron salt bid–qid	10–16 mg iron salt/kg day

Side Effects:
GI upset, nausea, vomiting, diarrhea, constipation, darkening of stools.
Liquid preparation may stain teeth.

Precautions:
Use chronically only in iron-deficient patients.
GI upset may be minimized by administering with meals and gradually increasing doses.

Contraindications:
Hemochromatosis, hemosiderosis, hemolytic anemias.
Iron may aggravate peptic ulcer disease, ulcerative colitis, or regional enteritis.

Drug Interactions:
Iron may decrease the GI absorption of tetracyclines and penicillamine.
Magnesium trisilicate and calcium carbonate may decrease iron absorption.
Vitamin C may increase the GI absorption of iron.

Monitor: Hemoglobin, hematocrit, reticulocyte count, Fe/TIBC, ferritin.

FLUOROURACIL (5-FU, Adrucil)

Pharmacologic Class: Antimetabolite antineoplastic.

Mechanism of Action: Inhibition of DNA synthesis by inhibiting thymidilate synthetase.

Indications: Used alone or in combination as an antineoplastic for carcinoma of breast, stomach, colon, rectum, and pancreas.

Route of Excretion: Metabolized by the liver, 10–15% excreted unchanged renally.

Dosage: 12 mg/kg/d IV × 4 days, then 6 mg/kg q other day × 4 doses. Repeat dose q 30 days after last dose or 10–15 mg/kg/wk, ≯ 1 g/wk.

Adverse Reactions: Alopecia, dermatitis, photosensitivity, nail loss; **anorexia, nausea, vomiting, diarrhea, stomatitis;** angina; **leukopenia** (9–25 days postdrug), **thrombocytopenia;** lethargy, acute cerebellar syndrome; fever.

Precautions: Use cautiously in patients with infections, bone marrow depression, poor nutritional status, and severe hepatic dysfunction.

Contraindications:
Hypersensitivity.
Avoid during pregnancy and lactation.

Drug Interactions: Additive bone marrow depression with radiation and other antineoplastics.

Monitor: CBC, oral mucosa.

FUROSEMIDE (Lasix)

Pharmacologic Class: Loop diuretic.

Mechanism of Action: Inhibits NaCl reabsorption in thick ascending loop of Henle.

Indications:
Edema due to congestive heart failure, hepatic disease, or renal disease.
Acute pulmonary edema.
Hypertension.
Hypercalcemia.

Pharmacodynamics:

	Onset	Peak	Duration
po	30–60 min	1–2 hr	6–8 hr
IM	10–30 min	1 hr	4–8 hr
IV	5 min	30 min	2 hr

Route of Excretion: Renal (66%), hepatic (34%).

Dosage:

	Initial	Maintenance	Maximum
Adult: po/IV/IM	20–80 mg daily (q AM)	Increase by 20–40 mg until desired response. Administer daily or BID	600 mg/d
Pediatric: po/IV/IM	2 mg/kg		6 mg/kg

(Note: Rate of administration should not exceed 4 mg/min, especially in renal failure and when using high doses.)
Dosage adjustment for renal failure: Higher doses (80–600 mg) may be required in end-stage renal disease.

Side Effects: Hypokalemia, hypochloremic metabolic alkalosis, **hyponatremia**, azotemia, **dehydration**, hypomagnesemia; ototoxicity; **hyperuricemia**, hyperglycemia; rash, photosensitivity; pancreatitis; nonocclusive intestinal infarction.

Precautions:
Digoxin and CHF—hypokalemia may increase risk of digoxin toxicity.
Hepatic failure—hypokalemia may precipitate hepatic encephalopathy and/or hepatorenal syndrome.
Increasing azotemia, oliguria: discontinue furosemide.

Contraindications: Avoid in hypersensitivity, pregnancy, and lactation.

Drug Interactions:
Increased digitalis toxicity due to hypokalemia.

Corticosteroids may increase risk of hypokalemia.
Increased furosemide effect by metolazone, clofibrate.
Decreased furosemide effect by NSAIDs, phenytoin.
Furosemide increases effect of antihypertensives, lithium, clofibrate, tubocurarine, salicylates, theophylline.
Furosemide decreases effect of norepinephrine.
Furosemide may increase risk of aminoglycoside atotoxicity.

Monitor: Serum electrolytes (Na^+, K^+, Cl^-, HCO_3^-, MG^{++}), BUN, creatinine, glucose, uric acid, weight, intake and output, blood pressure.

GENTAMICIN (Garamycin, Apogen, Bristagen)
(Other antibiotics with similar spectrum of action: tobramycin, netilmicin, amikacin)

Pharmacologic Class: Aminoglycoside antibiotic.

Mechanism of Action: Inhibition of bacterial protein synthesis.

Indications: Infections caused by susceptible organisms: *E. coli, Klebsiella, Proteus, Acinetobacter, Citrobacter, Enterobacter, Providencia, Pseudomonas* (may use in combination with anti-pseudomonal penicillin), *Salmonella, Serratia, Staphylococcus, Enterococcus* (used synergistically with a penicillin). Use topically for serious burn infections.

Pharmacokinetics: Minimal oral absorption, well absorbed following IM injection (peak 0.5–1.5 hr); renally excreted, t $1/2$ 2–5 hr; therapeutic gentamicin concentrations = 4–10 mcg/ml.

Dose: IM/IV: Adult, 3–5 mg/kg/d in 3 divided doses; pediatric, 6–7.5 mg/kg/d in 3 divided doses; premature infants and neonates, 5 mg/kg/d in 2 divided doses. Reduce dose with renal impairment.

Adverse Reactions: Ototoxicity (hearing loss and vestibular damage); **nephrotoxicity;** neuromuscular blockade; superinfection; allergic reactions.

Precautions: Narrow therapeutic-toxic ratio.

Contraindication: Hypersensitivity; cross-sensitivity with other aminoglycosides.

Drug Interactions:
Increased risk of toxicity when used concomitantly with other ototoxic and nephrotoxic agents and neuromuscular blockers.
In vitro inactivation may occur when aminoglycosides are mixed with penicillins and cephalosporins.

Monitor: WBC, temperature, culture and sensitivity, serum levels.

HALOPERIDOL (Haldol)

Pharmacologic Class: Butyrophenone antipsychotic.

Mechanism of Action: Block dopamine-2 receptors in the brain.

Indications:
Treatment of psychotic disorders.
Tourette's syndrome.
Severe behavioral disorders in children.
Antiemetic.

Route of Excretion: Primarily metabolized by the liver.

Dosage:
Oral
  Adult: 0.5–5.0 mg bid–tid, up to 100 mg/d
  Children: 0.05–0.15 mg/kg/d in 2–3 divided doses
IM: 2–5 mg, may repeat q 30–60 min prn, usually q 4–8 hr
IV: 2–25 mg q 30 minutes at a rate of 5 mg/min
Haloperidol decanoate IM: 10–15 times daily oral dose q 4 weeks.

Adverse Reactions: **Sedation,** depression, **extrapyramidal reactions,** tardive dyskinesias, seizures; **orthostatic hypotension,** tachycardia; rash, **photosensitivity;** impotence, gynecomastia, amenorrhea, galactorrhea; **dry mouth, weight gain, constipation,** hepatitis, urinary retention; blood dyscrasias; rash.

Precautions:
Use cautiously in elderly and in patients with prostatic hypertrophy, seizure disorder, glaucoma.
Tardive dyskinesias are most likely to develop in patient treated with high cumulative doses for long duration.
Drowsiness is greatest during first 2 weeks of therapy. Caution patients concerning driving and operating hazardous machinery.

Drug Interactions:
Lithuim may alter haloperidol response and vice versa. Potential increased neurotoxicity.
Haloperidol may inhibit metabolism of tricyclics.
Anticholinergics, methyldopa may impair response to haloperidol.
Haloperidol may antagonize effects of amphetamines.

Monitor: Symptomatic response; blood pressure, extrapyramidal reactions.

HEPARIN (Liquaemin, Calciparine)

Pharmacologic Class: Anticoagulant.

Mechanism of Action: Heparin increases the activity of antithrombin III, thus inactivating factor Xa, and prevents the conversion of prothrombin to thrombin. Large quantities also inactivate thrombin and prevent the conversion of fibrinogen to fibrin.

Indications:
Prophylaxis and treatment of thromboembolic disorders.
Treatment of disseminated intravascular coagulation.
Prevent clotting of blood in extracorporeal circulation.

Route of Excretion: Partially metabolized by the liver and the reticuloendothelial system; partial renal elimination; $t^1/_2$ 1–2.5 hr.

Dosage:
Individualize dose based upon PTT.
Adult
  IV bolus: 10,000 units (u), then 5000–10,000 u q 4–6 hr.
  IV infusion: 35–70 u/kg bolus, then 20,000–40,000 u/24 hr.
  SC: 10,000–20,000 u, then 8,000–10,000 u q 8 hr or 15,000–20,000 u q 12 hr.
  (prophylaxis) 5,000 u q 8–12 hr.
Children: 50 u/kg IV, then 100 u/kg IV q 4 hr or 20,000 u/m^2/24 hr.

Adverse Reactions: Bleeding, hemorrhage, **thrombocytopenia**, hematoma after SC injection; chills, fever; rash, alopecia; hepatitis; osteoporosis, hyperkalemia, hypoaldosteronism.

Precautions: Use cautiously in patients with renal or hepatic disease, history of peptic ulcer disease, hypertension, in last trimester of pregnancy, and immediately postpartum.

Contraindications: Uncontrolled bleeding, hemophilia, hypersensitivity.

Drug Interactions: Increased risk of bleeding with oral anticoagulants, aspirin, NSAIDs, dipyridamole, sulfinpyrazone, dextran, and thrombolytic therapy.

Monitor: PTT (therapeutic range 1.5–2 times control), CBC, stool for occult blood.

HYDRALAZINE (Apresoline)

Pharmacologic Class: Vasodilator.

Mechanism of Action: Direct-acting peripheral arteriolar vasodilation resulting in lowered blood pressure, decreased peripheral resistance (decreased afterload), and reflex tachycardia.

Indications:
Hypertension.
Congestive heart failure.

Pharmacodynamics:

	Onset	Peak	Duration
po	20–30 min	1–2 hr	6–12 hr
IM	10–30 min	1 hr	4–6 hr
IV	5–20 min	10–80 min	4–6 hr

Route of Excretion: Metabolized by the liver acetylation.

Dosage:
Oral
  Adults: 40–400 mg/d in 2–4 divided doses.
  Children: 0.75–7.5 mg/kg/d in 2–4 divided doses.
IM/IV
  Adults: 20–40 mg q 4–6 hr prn.
  Children: 0.1–0.2 mg/kg q 4–6 hr prn.

Adverse Reactions: Headache, dizziness, peripheral neuritis, depression, anxiety; **tachycardia, palpitations,** angina, hypotension, edema; **nausea,** vomiting, diarrhea; arthralgias, myalgias, **lupus-like reaction** (usually >400 mg/d); fever; blood dyscrasias.

Precautions: Use cautiously in patients with coronary artery cerebrovascular and severe renal disease.

Contraindications: Hypersensitivity, mitral valvular rheumatic heart disease, acute dissecting aortic aneurysm.

Drug interactions:
Additive hypotensive effect with nitrates and other antihypertensives, especially diazoxide and MAO inhibitors.
Additive chronotropic effect with sympathomimetics.

Monitor: Blood pressure, heart rate, ANA.

HYDROCHLOROTHIAZIDE (HCTZ, Esidrix, HydroDiuril, Oretic)

(Other similar agents: Chlorothiazide, benzthiazide, bendroflumethiazide, cyclothiazide, methyclothiazide, metolazone, quinethazone, chlorthalidone, indapamide)

Pharmacologic Class: Thiazide diuretic.

Mechanism of Action: Inhibition of NaCl reabsorption at the cortical diluting segment. Lowers blood pressue by direct arteriolar relaxation.

Indications:
Hypertension.
Edema due to congestive heart failure, hepatic or renal disease.
Nephrogenic diabetes insipidus.
Idiopathic hypercalciuria.

Pharmacodynamics:

	Onset	Peak	Duration
po (diuretic)	2 hr	4–6 hr	6–12 hr
po (antihypertensive)	3–4 d	7–14 d	7 d

Route of Excretion: Primarily excreted unchanged by kidneys.

Dosage:
Adult: 12.5–200 mg/d in 1–2 divided doses.
Children: >6 mo, 2.2 mg/kg in 2 divided doses; <6 mo, 3.3 mg/kg in 2 divided doses.

Adverse Reactions: Hypokalemic hypochloremic metabolic alkalosis, hyponatremia, dehydration, hypercalcemia, hypomagnesemia, hypophosphatemia, **hyperuricemia,** azotemia, hyperglycemia; rash, photosensitivity; hypotension; pancreatitis; blood dyscrasias (leukopenia, thrombocytopenia).

Precautions:
Patients with creatinine clearance less than 40 ml/min may not respond to HCTZ, or it may worsen their azotemia.
Thiazide-induced hypokalemia may precipitate hepatic coma in patients with cirrhosis.
Thiazide-induced hypokalemia may increase risk of digoxin toxicity.

Contraindications: Hypersensitivity; cross-reactivity with other sulfonamides—avoid in patients with serious sulfa allergy.

Drug Interactions:
Additive hypotension with nitrates or other antihypertensives. Colestipol and cholestyramine may decrease HCTZ absorption.
Increased risk of hypokalemia with amphotericin, aminoglycosides, corticosteroids, carbenicillin/ticarcillin.

HCTZ decreases lithium excretion and increases lithium levels.

Monitor: Blood pressure, heart rate, volume status; serum electrolytes (Na^+, K^+, Cl^-, HCO_3, Mg^{++}, Ca^{++}), BUN, creatinine, glucose, uric acid, weight, intake and output.

IBUPROFEN (Motrin, Advil, Nuprin)
(Other similar agents: fenoprofen, ketoprofen, naproxen)

Pharmacologic Class: Nonsteroidal anti-inflammatory agent, propionic-acid derivative.

Mechanism of Action: Inhibits prostaglandin synthesis.

Indications:
Rheumatoid arthritis and osteoarthritis.
Dysmenorrhea.
Analgesic.
Antipyretic.

Route of Excretion: Primarily metabolized by the liver; metabolites largely excreted through kidney.

Dosage: 200–800 mg tid–qid.

Adverse Reactions: Epigastric pain, nausea, vomiting, constipation, diarrhea, GI bleeding; **dizziness,** headache; hyperkalemia, edema, renal insufficiency, nephrotic syndrome; blood dyscrasias, prolonged bleeding time due to antiplatelet effect; rash.

Precautions: Use cautiously in elderly patients with severe cardiac or impaired renal function, history of peptic ulcer disease.

Contraindications: Hypersensitivity, may have cross-reactivity with other NSAIDs, active GI bleeding.

Drug Interactions:
May decrease response to loop and thiazide diuretics.
May increase serum digoxin concentrations in some patients.
Combination of ibuprofen and aspirin decreases net anti-inflammatory activity.

Monitor: Symptomatic response, hematocrit, stool for occult blood, renal function.

IMIPENEM/CILASTATIN (Primaxin)

Pharmacologic Class: Carbapenem antibiotic.

Mechanism of Action: Imipenem, a thienamycin antibiotic, inhibits cell-wall synthesis. Cilastatin inhibits dehydropeptidase I, preventing renal metabolism of imipenem.

Indications: Infections caused by susceptible organisms: *Staphylococcus, Streptococcus pneumoniae*, group A beta-hemolytic *Streptococcus*, group D streptococci; *E. coli, Proteus, Klebsiella, Serratia, Acinetobacter, Pseudomonas, Citrobacter*, anaerobes including *B. fragilis.*

Route of Excretion: 70% excreted renally, t$^{1/2}$ 1 hr.

Dosage: IV: 250–1000 mg q 6 hr. Reduce dose with renal impairment.

Adverse Reactions: Nausea, vomiting, diarrhea, hepatitis; blood hyscrasias; superinfection; fever, rash, phlebitis; seizures, dizziness.

Precautions: Use cautiously in patients with seizure disorder and history of multiple drug allergies.

Contraindications: Hypersensitivity; may have cross-sensitivity with penicillins and cephalosporins.

Drug interactions:
Probenecid increases blood levels of imipenem/cilastatin.
Do not administer with aminoglycosides *in vitro*.

Monitor: WBC, temperature, culture and sensitivity.

INDOMETHACIN (Indocin)
(Other similar agents: sulindac, tolmetin)

Pharmacologic Class: Nonsteroidal anti-inflammatory drugs, indole derivative.

Mechanism of Action: Inhibits prostaglandin synthesis.

Indications:
Rheumatoid arthritis; osteoarthritis, ankylosing spondylitis, acute gouty arthritis.
Analgesic; acute bursitis.
IV—closure of patent ductus arteriosus.

Pharmacodynamics: Onset 30 min, peak 0.5–2 hr, duration 6–12 hr.

Route of Excretion: Primarily metabolized by the liver.

Dosage: po/rectal 50–200 mg in 2–4 divided doses.

Adverse Reactions: Epigastric pain, nausea, vomiting, constipation, GI bleeding, hepatitis; **headache,** drowsiness, dizziness, tinnitus, edema, hyperkalemia, renal insufficiency, nephrotic syndrome; blood dyscrasias, prolonged bleeding time due to antiplatelet effect; rash.

Precautions: Use cautiously in elderly, patients with severe cardiac or impaired renal function, history of peptic ulcer disease.

Contraindications: Hypersensitivity, may have cross-sensitivity with other NSAIDs, active GI bleeding.

Drug Interactions:
May prolong PT in patients treated with oral anticoagulants.
May decrease response to loop and thiazide diuretics.
Combination of diflunisal and indomethacin increases indomethacin plasma levels and increases risk of toxicity.
Combination of indomethacin and triamterene may cause acute renal failure.
Indomethacin may inhibit captopril's response.
Combination of indomethacin and corticosteroids increases risk of GI ulceration.
Indomethacin decreases lithium excretion and increases plasma lithium levels.

Monitor: Symptomatic response, hematocrit, stool for occult blood, renal function.

INSULIN

Pharmacologic Class: Hormone.

Mechanism of Action: Lowers blood glucose by increasing intracellular conversion of glucose to glycogen.

Indications:
Diabetes mellitus.
Hyperkalemia.

Pharmacodynamics:

	Onset	Peak	Duration
Regular SC	0.5–1 hr	2–5 hr	5–8 hr
Regular IV	10–30 min	15–30 min	0.5–1.0 hr
Semilente SC	1-1.5 hr	4–10 hr	12–16 hr
NPH SC	1–2 hr	4–12 hr	18–28 hr
Lente SC	1–2.5 hr	7–15 hr	18–28 hr
PZI SC	4–8 hr	14–24 hr	36 hr
Ultralente SC	4–8 hr	10–30 hr	36 hr

Route of Excretion: Metabolized by liver, kidneys, and muscle.

Dosage: Individualize dose.

Adverse Reactions: Hypoglycemia, rebound hyperglycemia; redness, swelling, itching, lipodystrophy at injection sites, rash, angioedema, anaphylaxis.

Precautions: Increased insulin requirements during stress, infection, and pregnancy. Doses vary depending on diet and exercise and on amount of endogenous insulin available.

Contraindications: Hypersensitivity to animal products (beef or pork) may require change in animal source or to human insulin.

Drug Interactions:
Corticosteroids, ethanol, thiazide diuretics, oral contraceptives, thyroid preparations may increase insulin requirements.
Tricyclics, MAO inhibitors, anabolic steroids, ethanol, oxytetracycline, phenylbutazone, and salicylates may decrease insulin requirements.
Beta blockers may mask some symptoms of hypoglycemia and may prolong hypoglycemic episodes.

Monitor: Blood and urine glucose and ketones, serum potassium.

ISONIAZID (INH, Nydrazid, Laniazid)

Pharmacologic Class: Antitubercular agent.

Mechanism of Action: Unknown, probably inhibits cell-wall synthesis.

Indications: Prophylaxis and treatment of tuberculosis.

Route of Excretion: 50% acetylated by the liver, remainder excreted unchanged renally.

Dosage:
Adult: 5 mg/kg/d (maximum 300 mg/d) or 15 mg/kg 2–3 times weekly.
Children: 10–20 mg/kg/d or 20–40 mg/kg 2 times weekly.

Adverse Reactions: Peripheral neuropathy, seizures, psychoses, optic neuritis; nausea, vomiting, **hepatitis;** blood dyscrasias, fever, rash; hypocalcemia, hyperglycemia, gynecomastia.

Precautions:
Pyridoxine administration (6–50 mg/d) may decrease risk of peripheral neuropathy.
Increased risk of hepatitis with age >35 yr., chronic alcohol ingestion.
Monitor patients with active chronic liver disease and severe renal impairment.
Periodic ophthalmic examinations if visual symptoms occur.

Contraindications: Hypersensitivity, isoniazid hepatitis.

Drug Interactions:
INH may increase serum levels of carbamazepine. Carbamazepine may increase risk of INH-induced hepatotoxicity.
INH inhibits metabolism of phenytoin.
Aluminum hydroxide and magaldrate decrease GI absorption of INH. Enhanced hepatic metabolism of INH by corticosteroids. INH may decrease metabolism of corticosteroids.
Behavioral changes in patients treated concomitantly with INH and disulfiram.
Rifampin may increase hepatic metabolism of INH and increase risk of hepatotoxicity.

Monitor: LFTs, temperature, AFB, symptoms of peripheral neuropathy, visual changes.

ISOSORBIDE DINITRATE (ISDN, Isordil, Sorbitrate)

Pharmacologic Class: Coronary vasodilator nitrate.

Mechanism of Action: Relaxes vascular smooth muscle, producing vasodilation (veins > arteries). Dilates coronary arteries and improves collateral flow in ischemic myocardium. Reduces myocardial oxygen consumption. Dilates capacitance vessels, causing venous pooling and decreased left ventricular end diastolic pressure, decreased preload.

Indications:
Prophylaxis and treatment of angina.
Congestive heart failure.

Pharmacodynamics:

	Onset	Duration
Sublingual, chewable	2–5 min	0.5–2 hr
Oral	15–40 min	4 hr
Extended release	30 min	6–12 hr

Route of Excretion: Hepatically metabolized.

Dosage:
Sublingual: 2.5–10 mg q 4–6 hr and prn angina.
Chewable: 5–10 mg q 2–3 hr and prn angina.
Oral: 5–30 mg qid; ER: 40 mg q 6–12 hr.

Adverse Reactions: **Headache, dizziness,** syncope, apprehension, restlessness, weakness; **tachycardia, hypotension,** palpitations; abdominal pain, nausea, vomiting; **flushing,** rash; tolerance.

Precautions: Use cautiously in patients with head trauma or cerebral hemorrhage. Avoid extended release preparations in patients with GI hypermotility or malabsorption.

Contraindications: Hypersensitivity, severe anemia.

Drug Interactions: Additive hypotensive effects with calcium channel blockers, alcohol, beta blockers, antihypertensives, and phenothiazines.

Monitor: Blood pressure, heart rate, ECG, symptoms.

LABETOLOL (Normodyne, Trandate)

Pharmacologic Class: α_1 and β adrenoceptor antagonist.

Mechanism of Action: Due to α_1 and beta blockade, blood pressure is decreased without a reflex tachycardia.

Indication: Hypertension.

Pharmacodynamics:

	Onset	Peak	Duration
po	0.3–2 hr	1–4 hr	8–12 hr
IV	2–5 min	5–15 min	2–18 hr

Route of Excretion: Primarily hepatically metabolized.

Dosage:
Oral: 100 mg bid, increase by 100 mg bid q 2–3 days; maximum 2400 mg/d.
IV: 20 mg/2 min, give additional 40–80 mg q 10 min prn or 2 mg/min infusion. Maximum daily dose 300 mg.

Adverse Reactions: Postural hypotension, bradycardia, CHF; bronchospasm; **fatigue,** headache; nausea, diarrhea, jaundice; impotence; muscle cramps, dry eyes; lupus-like syndrome; flushing, rash.

Precautions:
Use cautiously with impaired hepatic function, CHF.
Labetolol may mask symptoms of hypoglycemia and thyrotoxicosis.
Administer IV labetolol to supine patients.

Contraindications: Asthma, uncompensated CHF, greater than first-degree AV heart block, severe bradycardia, cardiogenic shock.

Drug Interactions:
Labetolol may antagonize effect of beta-adrenergic agonists.
Additive hypotensive effect with nitrates, halothane, or other antihypertensives.
Additive bradycardia with digoxin.
Cimetidine may decrease labetolol's bioavailability.
Labetolol concomitantly with tricyclics increases the incidence of tremors.

Monitor: Blood pressure, heart rate.

LEVODOPA/CARBIDOPA (Sinemet)

Pharmacologic Class: Antiparkinson agent.

Mechanism of Action: Levodopa is a precursor to dopamine, which crosses the blood-brain barrier, to restore deficient dopamine levels in the striatum. Carbidopa inhibits the peripheral decarboxylation of levodopa.

Indication: Treatment of parkinsonism.

Route of Excretion: Levodopa is metabolized by the liver and GI tract; carbidopa is excreted unchanged by the kidneys (30%).

Dosage: Carbidopa/levodopa 75/300–200/2000 mg/d in 3–4 divided doses (tablets: 10/100, 25/100, 25/250).

Adverse Reactions: Drooling, dry mouth, dysguesia; **anorexia, nausea, vomiting,** abdominal pain, diarrhea, constipation; **abnormal involuntary movements, tremor, ataxia,** memory loss, mental changes, dizziness; palpitations, postural hypotension; blood dyscrasia; azotemia; hepatitis; rash; blurred vision.

Precautions: Use cautiously in patients with wide-angle glaucoma; severe cardiovascular, pulmonary, cerebrovascular, renal, hepatic, endocrine, psychiatric, or ulcer disease.

Contraindications: Hypersensitivity, MAO inhibitors, narrow-angle glaucoma, malignant melanoma, or suspicious skin lesions.

Drug Interactions:
Decrease efficacy of levodopa with phenytoin, reserpine, clonidine, antipsychotics, benzodiazepines, papaverine, pyridoxine (not if patient also treated with carbidopa).
Increased blood pressure in patients treated with MAO inhibitors.
Increased postural hypotension with tricyclics, methyldopa, diuretics, and guanethidine.
Anticholinergics may decrease GI absorption of levodopa.

Monitor: Blood pressure, symptomatic relief, CNS and GI toxicity.

LEVOTHYROXINE (T$_4$, Synthroid, Levothroid)

Pharmacologic Class: Thyroid hormone.

Mechanism of Action: Increases the metabolic rate of body tissues.

Indication:
Hypothyroidism.
Treatment or prevention of euthyroid goiter.

Route of Excretion: Metabolized by the liver, biliary excretion.

Dosage:
Oral
  Adult: 0.1–0.4 mg/day; initiate therapy at 0.025–0.050 mg/d, increase dose every 2–4 weeks.
  Pediatric (>12 yr) 2–3 mcg/kg/d; (1–12 yr) 4–6 mcg/kg/d; (<1 yr) 6–10 mcg/kg/d.
IV
  Give 50–80% of oral dose for replacement therapy in NPO patient; myxedema coma 0.2–0.5 mg on day 1, additional 0.1–0.3 mg on second day of treatment.

Adverse Reactions: Tremors, nervousness, headache, insomnia; tachycardia, palpitations, angina, hypertension; diarrhea, nausea, vomiting; weight loss, sweating, heat intolerance, fever (adverse reactions are rare except for overdosage).

Precautions:
Use cautiously in patients with cardiovascular disease, elderly and myxedematous patients.
Initiate treatment of low doses and increase dose slowly.
Thyroid hormones aggravate symptoms in patients with diabetes mellitus, diabetes insipidus, and adrenal insufficiency.

Contraindications:
Acute myocardial infarction, thyrotoxicosis, untreated adrenal insufficiency.

Drug Interactions:
Thyroid hormones increase effect of oral anticoagulants. Reduce warfarin dose when thyroid is added.
Phenytoin increases metabolism of thyroid hormones.
Thyroid hormones may increase dose requirement of insulin and oral hypoglycemics.
Cholestyramine decreases the GI absorption of levothyroxine.

Monitor: T$_4$, T$_3$, TSH; blood pressure, heart rate.

LIDOCAINE (Xylocaine)

Pharmacologic Class: Type I antiarrhythmic, sodium channel depressor.

Mechanism of Action: Suppresses automaticity in ventricles; membrane stabilizer.

Indications: Ventricular arrhythmias; topically, as local anesthetic.

Route of Excretion: Metabolized by liver to two active metabolites which are renally eliminated.

Dosage:
Pediatric and Adult: IV bolus 1 mg/kg, may repeat $1/3$–$1/2$ dose if no response in 5 minutes; then continuous infusion (20–50 mcg/kg/min).
Adult—IM (only if unable to give IV): (4.3 mg/kg), may repeat in 60–90 minutes.
Reduce dose with CHF, liver disease, age >60 yr.
Topically, 4% solution, 1–5 ml.

Adverse Reactions: Drowsiness, paresthesias, tremors, seizures, dizziness, respiratory depression; hypotension, bradycardia, arrest; uticaria.

Precautions:
Reduced doses in elderly (>60 yr), CHF, liver disease.
Use cautiously with bradycardia or heart block, severe digitalis intoxication, renal failure.
Lidocaine may precipitate malignant hyperthermic crisis.

Contraindications: Hypersensitivity; severe SA, AV, or intraventricular heart block, Adams-Stokes or Wolff-Parkinson-White syndromes.

Drug Interactions:
Beta blockers and cimetidine may inhibit metabolism of lidocaine. Phenytoin may increase metabolism of lidocaine and increase cardiac depressant effect.
Lidocaine may increase neuromuscular blockade of skeletal muscle relaxants: tubocurarine, neomycin, polymyxin B.

Monitor: ECG, blood pressure, heart rate, serum lidocaine 1.5–5.0 mcg/ml.

LITHIUM
(L. Carbonate—Eskalith, Lithane, Lithonate, Lithobid;
L. Citrate—Cibalith S)

Pharmacologic Class: Antimanic agent.

Mechanism of Action: Alters sodium transport and uptake of neurotransmitters.

Indications:
Bipolar affective disorders.
Prophylaxis of cluster and migraine headaches.
Chemotherapy-induced neutropenia.

Route of Excretion: Primarily excreted unchanged by kidneys, $t^{1/2}$ 20–27 hr.

Dosage: Adjust dose to trough serum lithium = 0.6–1.2 mEq/Liter and clinical response; 0.9–1.8 g/day in 3–4 divided doses, extended release forms given bid.

Adverse Reactions: **Tremor, headache,** lethargy, fatigue, twitching, ataxia, dizziness, slurred speech, restlessness, confusion, stupor, coma; arrhythmia, hypotension; anorexia, nausea, vomiting, diarrhea, flatulence, dysgeusia, dry mouth; polyuria, nephrogenic diabetes insipidus, chronic interstitial nephritis; muscle weakness; **hypothyroidism, goiter, weight gain;** leukocytosis; rash.

Precautions:
Monitor blood levels carefully—narrow toxic-therapeutic ratio.
Avoid sodium depletion. Maintain normal salt and fluid intake.

Contraindications: Severe cardiovascular or renal disease.

Drug Interactions:
Diuretics, indomethacin, piroxicam, and decreased sodium chloride intake increase lithium concentrations.
Theophylline, sodium bicarbonate, increased sodium chloride intake decrease lithium concentrations.
Increased neurotoxicity with carbamazepine, methyldopa, phenothiazines, and haloperidol.
Increased hypothyroid activity with potassium iodide.
Lithium may prolong neuromuscular blockade of succinylcholine.

Monitor: Serum lithium concentrations (therapeutic = 0.6–1.2 mEq/Liter), thyroid function tests, renal function.

MEPERIDINE (Demerol)

Pharmacologic Class: Opioid analgesic.

Mechanism of Action: Binds to CNS opiate receptors and alters response to pain. Produces CNS depression.

Indications:
Moderate to severe pain.
Preoperative sedation.
Limited analgesia (e.g., obstetrics—reduced respiratory depression in fetus).

Route of Excretion: Metabolized by the liver to normeperidine, an eliptogenic metabolite which accumulates with renal failure.

Dosage:
Adult: IM/SC/po 50–150 mg q 3–4 hr prn.
Children: IM/SC/po 1–1.8 mg/kg q 3–4 hr prn.

Adverse Reactions: Sedation, dizziness, lightheadedness, dysphoria, confusion, hallucinations, seizures, respiratory depression; **nausea, vomiting, constipation,** dry mouth; **hypotension,** arrhythmias, cardiac arrest; urinary retention; blurred vision; allergic reaction; physical or psychological dependence.

Precautions:
Use cautiously in elderly and patients with severe renal disease, seizure disorder, acute abdomen, head trauma, increased intracranial pressure, alcoholism, pulmonary disease, prostatic hypertrophy, liver disease.
Warn patients about sedation when driving and operating hazardous machinery.

Contraindications: Hypersensitivity, respiratory depression, acute asthmatic attack.

Drug Interactions:
Additive CNS depression with alcohol, antihistamines, barbiturates, benzodiazepines, sedative/hypnotic, antidepressants, antipsychotics, and general anesthetics.
Severe reactions in patients treated with MAO inhibitors.
Barbiturates may increase metabolism of meperidine, resulting in increased normeperidine concentrations.

Monitor: Pain relief, respirations, blood pressure.

METAPROTERENOL (Alupent, Metaprel)

Pharmacologic Class: Beta-adrenergic agonist.

Mechanism of Action: Beta-adrenergic agonist stimulates adenyl cyclase and increases cyclic AMP concentrations producing bronchodilation.

Indications: Bronchodilator for asthma or COPD.

Route of Excretion: Metabolized by the liver.

Dosage:
Oral
  Adult: 20 mg tid–qid.
  Pediatric: (<9 yr) 10 mg tid–qid.
Metered dose inhaler: 2–3 inhalations q 3–4 hr.
Hand-held nebulizer: 5–15 inhalations tid–qid.
IPPB 0.2–0.3 ml of 5% sol or 2.5 ml of 0.6% sol tid–qid.

Adverse Reactions: Tremor, nervousness, restlessness, dizziness, headache, insomnia; **palpitations, tachycardia,** hypertension, angina; nausea, vomiting, hyperglycemia.

Precautions:
Use cautiously in pregnant patients (may delay or stop labor) and in patients with diabetes, cardiac disease, hyperthyroidism, glaucoma, seizure disorder.
Tolerance or bronchospasm may develop with repeated use of inhalers.

Contraindications: Hypersensitivity, tachyarrhythmias.

Drug Interactions:
Routine administration of other sympathomimetic agents increase risk of tachycardia and hypertension.
Beta blockers may inhibit therapeutic effect.
Hypertensive crisis may occur in patients treated with MAO inhibitors.

Monitor: Respirations, heart rate, blood pressure.

METHADONE (Dolophine)

Pharmacologic Class: Opioid analgesic.

Mechanism of Action: Binds to CNS opiate receptors and alters response to pain. Produces CNS depression.

Indications:
Severe pain.
Detoxification/maintenance for heroin or narcotic analgesic addiction.

Pharmacodynamics:

	Onset	Peak	Duration
po	30–60 min	90–120 min	4–12 hr
IM/SC	10–20 min	60–120 min	4–6 hr

Route of Excretion: Metabolized by the liver.

Dosage:
Analgesia: 2.5–10 mg q 3–4 hr, up to 5–20 mg q 6–8 hr prn.
Detoxification: 15–40 mg/d.
Maintenance: 20–120 mg/d.

Adverse Reactions: Sedation, dizziness, lightheadedness, dysphoria, confusion, hallucinations, respiratory depression; **nausea, vomiting, constipation,** dry mouth; **hypotension,** arrhythmias, cardiac arrest; urinary retention; blurred vision; allergic reaction; physical or psychological dependence.

Precautions:
Use cautiously in patients with acute abdomen, head trauma, increased intracranial pressure, pulmonary disease.
Warn patients about sedation when driving and operating hazardous machinery.

Contraindications: Hypersensitivity, respiratory depression, acute asthmatic attack.

Drug Interactions:
Increased metabolism of methadone by rifampin, phenytoin.
Decreased metabolism of methadone by cimetidine.
Additive CNS depression with alcohol, sedative/hypnotic, antidepressants, antipsychotics, and general anesthetics.

Monitor: Pain, relief, respirations, blood pressure.

METHOTREXATE (MTX, Amethopterin, Folex, Mexate)

Pharmacologic Class: Antimetabolite neoplastic; immunosuppressant.

Mechanism of Action: Interferes with DNA synthesis by inhibiting folic acid reductase and preventing the formation of tetrahydrofolic acid.

Indications:
Used alone or in combination as an antineoplastic for acute lymphocytic leukemia; lymphosarcoma; mycosis fungoides; trophoblastic neoplasms; carcinoma of breast, lung (squamous and small cell), head, and neck.
Severe psoriasis.
Immunosuppressant to treat chronic rheumatoid arthritis, SLE, Wegener's granulomatosis.

Route of Excretion: Excreted unchanged by the kidneys.

Dosage: Varies greatly, depending on neoplasm:
Leukemia: induction, 3.3 mg/m^2/d for 4–6 wk; remission, 30 mg/m^2 po/IM twice weekly or 2.5 mg/kg IV q 14 d.
Lymphomas: 10–25 mg/d po for 4–8 d, rest 7–10 d, then repeat several courses; lymphosarcomas: 0.625–2.5 mg/kg/d.
Mycosis funcoides: 2.5–10 mg/d × wk or mo, 50 mg IM/wk, or 25 mg IM twice weekly.
Trophoblastic neoplasms: 15–30 mg/d po/IM for 5 days, repeat q wk × 3–5 courses.
Psoriasis: 7.5–25 mg oral/IM/IV q week.
Meningeal leukemia: 12 mg/m^2 or 15 mg intrathecally.

Adverse Reactions: Alopecia, rashes, acne, photosensitivity, depigmentation; anorexia, **nausea, vomiting,** diarrhea, **abdominal pain, stomatitis,** hematemesis, melena, hepatotoxicity; nephrotoxicity, hyperuricemia; bone marrow depression (**leukopenia,** anemia, thrombocytopenia); fever, infections; **malaise, fatigue, dizziness,** headaches, blurred vision, seizures; IT use: arachnoiditis, transient paresis, leukoencephalopathy.

Precautions:
Use cautiously in patients with infections, bone marrow suppression, impaired renal function, women of childbearing potential, peptic ulcer disease or ulcerative colitis. Leucovorin (citrovorum factor), reduced form of folate, may neutralize toxic hematopoietic effect.

Contraindications: Avoid during pregnancy, lactation, and in hypersensitive patients.

Drug Interactions:
Increased free MTX due to displacement from plasma proteins by

PABA, phenylbutazone, sulfonamides, salicylates, phenytoin, tetracycline, chloramphenicol.
Increased MTX concentrations due to impaired renal secretion by salicylates, probenecids, phenylbutazone, large-dose penicillins.
Pyrimethamine may increase MTX toxicity due to similar mechanism folic acid may decrease response to MTX.
Impairs response to vaccines.
Vincristine enhances cellular uptake of MTX.

Monitor: CBC, renal and liver functions, urinalysis, chest x-ray.

α-METHYLDOPA (Aldomet)

Pharmacologic Class: Centrally acting adrenergic agent.

Mechanism of Action: Stimulates central alpha-adrenergic receptors, false neurotransmission, and reduces plasma renin activity.

Indications: Hypertension.

Route of Excretion: Metabolized by liver to active metabolite; metabolite and unchanged drug excreted by kidneys.

Dosage:
Oral
  Adult: 500–3000 mg/d in 2–4 divided doses.
  Children: 10–65 mg/kg/d in 2–4 divided doses.
IV
  Adult: 250–1000 mg q 6 hr.
  Children 5–10 mg/kg q 6 hr.
Reduced dose with renal disease.

Adverse Reactions: Sedation, dizziness, headache, depression, decreased mental activity; **postural hypotension,** bradycardia, angina, myocarditis, weight gain, edema; nausea, vomiting, dry mouth, hepatitis, pancreatitis; **impotence,** gynecomastia; Coomb's positivity, hemolytic anemia, leukopenia, lupus-like syndrome; fever; nasal stuffiness.

Precautions: Use cautiously in patients with liver and renal disease.

Contraindications: Hypersensitivity, previous methyldopa hepatitis, active liver disease.

Drug Interactions:
Amphetamines, tricyclics, and phenothiazines may decrease methyldopa effect.
Additive CNS toxicity with haloperidol, levodopa, and lithium carbonate.
Additive hypotensive effect with nitrates, other antihypertensives, anesthetics, and levodopa.

Monitor: Blood pressure, liver function tests.

METOCLOPRAMIDE (Reglan)

Pharmacologic Class: Dopamine antagonist; GI stimulant.

Mechanism of Action: Stimulates motility of upper GI tract, relaxes pyloric sphincter, accelerates gastric emptying. Dopamine receptor antagonist in CNS.

Indications:
Diabetic gastroparesis.
Gastroesophageal reflux.
Antiemetic for chemotherapy-induced emesis.
Facilitate small-bowel intubation.
Facilitate radiographic exam of upper GI tract.

Route of Excretion: Primarily excreted in urine as unchanged drug (25%) or metabolites.

Dosage:
Gastroparesis/GE reflux: 10–15 mg qid (ac + hs).
Antiemetic: 1–2 mg/kg IV.
Radiologic exam and small bowel intubation; IV: adult: 10 mg; child: 6–14 yr, 2.5–5.0 mg; <6 yr, 0.1 mg/kg.

Adverse Reactions: Restlessness, drowsiness, fatigue, extrapyramidal reactions, dizziness, depression; **nausea, diarrhea;** hypertension, tachycardia.

Precautions:
Higher incidence of extrapyramidal reactions in children and elderly.
Warn patients about sedation when driving and operating hazardous machinery.

Contraindications: Hypersensitivity; patients with mechanical obstruction, seizure disorder, or pheochromocytoma.

Drug Interactions:
Effects antagonized by anticholinergics and narcotic analgesics. Decreases GI absorption of digoxin, cimetidine.
May increase GI absorption of acetaminophen, levodopa, tetracycline, ethanol.
Diabetics may require insulin dose adjustment.
Additive sedative effects with alcohol, narcotics, sedative/hypnotics.
May increase risk of extrapyramidal reactions with haloperidol or phenothiazines.

Monitor: Symptomatic relief, extrapyramidal reactions.

MILK OF MAGNESIA (Magnesium Hydroxide, MOM)

Pharmacologic Class: Nonsystemic-nonbuffer antacid; cathartic in large doses.

Mechanism of Action: Osmotically active in the lumen of the GI tract, attracts and retains water in intestinal lumen. Stimulates release of CCK, which stimulates motility of GI tract.

Indication: Laxative.

Route of Excretion: Magnesium which is absorbed is excreted by the kidneys.

Dosage:
Adult: 30–60 ml; children: 6–12 yr, 15–30 ml; 2–5 yr, 5–15 ml.

Side Effects: Diarrhea, abdominal cramps; weakness, dizziness, flushing, sweating; hypermagnesemia causing drowsiness, decreased deep tendon reflexes, bradycardia, hypotension.

Contraindications: Hypermagnesemia, hypocalcemia, severe renal failure (Cr Cl <25 ml/min), heart block.

Drug Interactions: Magnesium may potentiate neuromuscular blocking agents.

Monitor: Bowel movements; renal function; serum magnesium.

MINOXIDIL (Loniten)

Pharmacologic Class: Vasodilator antihypertensive agent.

Mechanism of Action: Acts as direct peripheral vasodilator on arterioles greater than veins, resulting in decreased blood pressure.

Indications:
Severe hypertension.
Fatigue due to low left ventricular output of CHF.
Topically—for treatment of male pattern baldness or alopecia areata.

Route of Excretion: 90% metabolized by the liver.

Dosage:
Adult: 5–100 mg/day in 1–2 divided doses.
Pediatric: <12 yr, 0.2–1.0 mg/kg/d.

Adverse Reactions: Headache; tachycardia, edema, CHF ECG changes, **sodium and water retention,** pericardial effusion and tamponade; nausea, vomiting, LFT changes; breast tenderness; rash, **hypertrichosis,** darkening of skin.

Precautions:
Administer minoxidil with a loop diuretic to prevent fluid retention; administration of a beta blocker or sympathetic blocking agent prevents reflex tachycardia.
Use cautiously in patients who have had recent myocardial infarction (<1 mo) and with severe renal impairment.

Contraindications: Hypersensitivity, pheochromocytoma, dissecting aortic aneurysm, acute MI.

Drug Interactions: Profound orthostatic hypotension when used with guanethidine.

Monitor: Blood pressure, weight, heart rate, edema.

MORPHINE SULFATE (Roxanol, MSIR)

Pharmacologic Class: Opioid analgesic.

Mechanism of Action: Binds to CNS opiate receptors and alters response to pain. Produces CNS depression.

Indications:
Moderate to severe pain.
Preoperative sedation.
Dyspnea with pulmonary edema.

Route of Excretion: Metabolized by the liver; increased sensitivity in renal failure patients due to alterations in protein binding or metabolites.

Dosage:
Adult
  Oral: 10–75 mg q 4 hr prn.
  Rectal: 10–20 mg q 4 hr prn.
  IM/SC: 5–20 mg q 4 hr prn.
  IV: 2.5–30 mg q 4 hr prn or infusion at 1–150 mg/hr.
Pediatric
  SC: 0.1–0.2 mg/kg q 4 hr prn.

Adverse Reactions: Sedation, dizziness, lightheadedness, dysphoria, confusion, hallucinations, respiratory depression; **nausea, vomiting, constipation,** dry mouth; hypotension, arrhythmias, cardiac arrest; urinary retention; blurred vision; depression of gonadotropin secretion; allergic reaction; physical or psychological dependence.

Precautions:
Use cautiously in elderly and in patients with severe renal disease, seizure disorder, acute abdomen, head trauma, increased intracranial pressure, alcoholism, pulmonary disease, prostatic hypertrophy.
Warn patients about sedation when driving and operating hazardous machinery.

Contraindications: Hypersensitivity, respiratory depression, acute asthmatic attack.

Drug Interactions:
Additive CNS depression with alcohol, antihistamines, barbiturates, benzodiazepines, sedatives/hypnotics, antidepressants, antipsychotics, and general anesthetics.
Severe reactions in patients treated with MAO inhibitors.
Naloxone antagonizes actions of morphine.

Monitor: Pain relief, respirations, blood pressure.

NAFCILLIN (Unipen)
(Other antibiotics with similar spectrum of action: cloxacillin, dicloxacillin, methicillin, oxacillin)

Pharmacologic Class: Penicillinase-resistant penicillin antibiotic.

Mechanism of Action: Bactericidal effect due to inhibition of synthesis of cell-wall mucopeptide.

Indications: Infections caused by susceptible organisms: penicillinase-producing *Staphylococcus aureus, Staphylococcus epidermidis, Streptococcus pneumoniae,* beta-hemolytic streptococci, *Streptococcus viridans.*

Route of Excretion: Hepatic inactivation, biliary secretion.

Dosage:
Adults: IV, 500–2000 mg q 4 hr; IM, 500 mg q 4–6 hr; po, 250–1000 mg q 4–6 hr.
Pediatric: IV, 50–200 mg/kg/d in 4–6 divided doses; IM, 25 mg/kg q 12 hr (neonates 10 mg/kg q 12 hr); po 25–50 mg/kg in 4 divided doses.

Adverse Reactions: Rash, allergic reactions, anaphylaxis; nausea, vomiting, diarrhea, pseudomembranous colitis, hepatitis; seizures; blood dyscrasias (granulocytopenia), bleeding abnormalities; phlebitis, tissue necrosis.

Precautions: Use cautiously in patient with impaired hepatic function. Do not use in patients with methicillin resistant infections.

Contraindications: Hypersensitivity to penicillin or cephalosporins.

Drug Interactions:
Activity of penicillins may be diminished when used concomitantly with bacteriostatic antibiotics (e.g., tetracyclines).
Do not admix nafcillin with aminoglycosides in IV bottle.

Monitor: Temperature, WBC, culture and sensitivity.

NIFEDIPINE (Adalat, Procardia)

Pharmacologic Class: Calcium channel antagonist, coronary vasodilator.

Mechanism of Action: Coronary vasodilation due to inhibition of calcium entry into vascular and myocardial smooth muscle.

Indications:
Angina pectoris.
Hypertension.
Severe, chronic CHF.

Route of Excretion: Primarily metabolized by the liver, duration 6–8 hr.

Dosage: 30–180 mg/d in 3–4 divided doses.

Adverse Reactions: Edema, rash; **dizziness, lightheadedness, headache,** weakness; **hypotension, palpitations,** CHF, pulmonary edema; **nausea;** hepatitis.

Precautions:
Rarely, patients treated with beta blockers and nifedipine may develop CHF.
Patients with angina may have an increase in frequency or severity of chest pain with initiation of nifedipine.
Use cautiously in patients with severe liver disease, CHF, edema.

Contraindications: Hypersensitivity.

Drug Interactions:
Increase in digoxin level.
Decrease in quinidine level.
Severe hypotension with fentanyl.

Monitor: Blood pressure, heart rate, edema, weight.

NITROFURANTOIN (Furadantin, Nitrofuran, Macrodantin)

Pharmacologic Class: Nitrofuran antibiotic.

Mechanism of Action: Interferes with acetyl CoA and inhibits bacterial carbohydrate metabolism.

Indication: Infections (especially of the urinary tract) caused by susceptible organisms: *E. Coli,* some *Klebsiella,* some *Enterobacter, Citrobacter, Enterococci,* group B streptococci, *Staphylococcus aureus, Staphylococcus epidermidis.*

Route of Excretion: 50% renally eliminated, t½ 20 min.

Dosage:
Adult: 100–400 mg/d in 4 divided doses; suppression 25–50 mg qid or 50–100 mg hs.
Pediatric: 5–7 mg/kg/d in 4 divided doses.
Reduced dose with renal dysfunction.

Adverse Reactions: Anorexia, nausea, vomiting (less frequent with macrocrystals), diarrhea, hepatitis, abdominal pain; peripheral neuropathy, headache, drowsiness, dizziness, nystagmus; photosensitivity, fever, rash; asthmatic attack, pulmonary fibrosis, pneumonitis; hemolytic anemia (especially with G-6-PD deficiency), blood dyscrasias.

Precautions:
Pneumonitis: acute—after 1–3 wk of therapy—dyspnea, chest pain, cough, fever, abnormal chest x-ray; chronic—after 1–6 mo of therapy.
Irreversible peripheral neuropathy—predisposing factors: renal insufficiency, anemia, diabetes, pyridoxine deficiency.
Risk of *Pseudomonas* superinfection.

Contraindications: Renal failure (CrCl <40 ml/min), pregnancy, infants <1 mo, hypersensitivity.

Drug Interactions:
Increased bioavailability with anticholinergic drugs.
Decreased bioavailability with magnesium trisilicate.

Monitor: WBC, temperature, culture and sensitivity.

NITROGLYCERIN (Nitrostat, Nitrobid, Nitrospan, Nitro Dur, Transderm-Nitro, Nitrodisc)

Pharmacologic Class: Coronary vasodilator.

Mechanism of Action: Relaxation of vascular smooth muscle, especially veins. Decrease left ventricular end-diastolic pressure (preload). Decrease blood pressure; decrease myocardial consumption. Improved coronary collateral flow.

Indications:
Prevention and treatment of anginal attacks.
Perioperative hypertension.
CHF.

Pharmacodynamics:

	Onset	**Duration**
IV	Immediate	2–5 minutes
Sublingual	1–3 min	30 min
Oral sustained release	40–60 min	4–8 hr
Ointment	20–60 min	2–12 hr
Transdermal patch	40–60 min	18–24 hr

Route of Excretion: Metabolized by the liver, $t^{1/2}$ 1–4 min.

Dosage: sl, 0.2–0.6 mg prn; oral, 2.5–26 mg tid–qid; ointment, 0.5–5 inches q 4 hr; patch 2.5–15 mg/d.

Adverse Reactions: Headache, dizziness, apprehension; **postural hypotension, tachycardia,** palpitations, syncope; nausea, vomiting; flushing, rash, tolerance.

Precautions:
Use cautiously in patients with head trauma or cerebral hemorrhage.
Tolerance to nitrates may develop—most likely with high doses over long time.
Use IV NTG cautiously in patients with liver and renal disease.
Remove transdermal patches before cardioversion.
Chest pain may be worsened in patients with hypertrophic cardiomyopathy.
IV NTG may adhere to plastics.
Concentration and release rate of topical preparations vary with manufacturer.

Contraindications: Hypotension, hypovolemia, severe anemia, hypersensitivity.

Drug Interactions:
Additive hypotension with alcohol, beta blockers, calcium channel blockers, phenothiazines, and antihypertensive drugs.
Smoking reduces effect on angina.

Monitor: Blood pressure (postural), heart rate, relief and frequency of symptoms.

NITROPRUSSIDE (Nipride, Nitropress)

Pharmacologic Class: Vasodilator.

Mechanism of Action: Direct peripheral vasodilation of arteries and veins, resulting in decreased blood pressure, increased cardiac output.

Indications:
Hypertensive crises.
Controlled hypotension during anesthesia.
CHF, cardiogenic shock.

Route of Excretion: Metabolized by RBCs and tissues to cyanide, then metabolized by liver to thiocyanate, which is renally excreted.

Dosage: 0.5–10 mcg/kg/min by IV infusion.

Adverse Reactions: Headache, dizziness, restlessness, apprehension; **nausea,** vomiting, abdominal pain; hypotension, palpitations, chest pain, dyspnea; muscle twitching; phlebitis.

Precautions:
Excess dose can produce cyanide toxicity (hypotension, metabolic acidosis, dyspnea, ataxia, headache, vomiting, diminished reflexes, coma).
Use cautiously with renal disease; discontinue if metabolic acidosis develops or thiocyanate toxicity (tinnitus, blurred vision, delirium).
Use cautiously with liver disease; cyanide may accumulate.

Contraindications: Decreased cerebral perfusion, coarctation of aorta, AV shunt leading to hypertension.

Drug Interactions: Additive hypotension with anesthetics, ganglionic blocking agents, and antihypertensive medications.

Monitor: Blood pressure, heart rate, thiocyanate levels, renal function, acid-base balance.

NORFLOXACIN (Noroxin)

Pharmacologic Class: Fluoroquinolone antibiotic.

Mechanism of Action: Inhibition of DNA synthesis probably by inhibiting bacterial DNA gyrase.

Indications: Infections (especially of the urinary tract) due to susceptible organisms: *E. coli, Enterobacter, Proteus, Serratia, Citrobacter, Klebsiella, Pseudomonas, H. influenzae, Neisseria, Staphylococcus aureus, Enterococci.*

Route of Excretion: Primarily renally eliminated, $t^{1}/_{2}$ 3–7 hours.

Dosage: 400 mg po bid. Reduced dose with severe renal disease.

Adverse Reactions: Dry mouth, dysgeusia, **nausea**, vomiting, anorexia, hepatitis; **dizziness, headache**, drowsiness, depression; neutropenia; allergic reaction.

Precautions: Advise patient to increase fluid intake and to take norfloxacin on an empty stomach and not concomitantly with antacids.

Contraindications: Hypersensitivity to norfloxacin, nalidixic acid, cinoxacin, ciprofloxacin.

Drug Interactions:
Decreased renal excretion with probenecid.
Nitrofurantoin may antagonize effect of norfloxacin.
Antacids may decrease GI absorption.

Monitor: Temperature, WBC, culture and sensitivity.

NYSTATIN (Mycostatin, Nilstat)

Pharmacologic Class: Antifungal.

Mechanism of Action: Change in membrane permeability of fungal cell by binding to sterols in cell membrane.

Indication: Oral candidiasis; use in other dosage forms for treatment of local Candida infections.

Route of Excretion: Poorly absorbed, excreted fecally.

Dosage:
Adults, children: 400,000–600,000 units q 6–8 hr.
Infants: 200,000 units q 6–8 hr.
Vaginal tablets: 1–2 times daily.

Adverse Reactions: Nausea, vomiting, diarrhea, abdominal upset.

Precautions: Vaginal tablets may be administered orally.

Contraindications: Hypersensitivity.

OXYCODONE (With acetaminophen in Percocet, Tylox; with aspirin in Percodan, Percodan-Demi)

Pharmacologic Class: Opioid analgesic.

Mechanism of Action: Binds to CNS opiate receptors and alters response to pain. Produces CNS depression.

Indications: Moderate to severe pain.

Route of Excretion: Metabolized by the liver, t$^{1}/_{2}$ 2–3 hr.

Dosage:
Adult: 5 mg q 6 hr prn.
Pediatric: (>12 yr) 2.5 mg q 6 hr prn; (6–12 yr) 1.25 mg q 6 hr prn.

Adverse Reactions: Sedation, dizziness, lightheadedness, dysphoria, confusion, hallucinations, respiratory depression; **nausea, vomiting, constipation,** dry mouth; hypotension, arrhythmias, cardiac arrest; urinary retention; blurred vision; allergic reaction; physical or psychological dependence.

Precautions:
Use cautiously in elderly, patients with severe renal disease, acute abdomen, head trauma, increased intracranial pressure, alcoholism, pulmonary disease, prostatic hypertrophy.
Warn patients about sedation when driving and operating hazardous machinery.

Contraindications: Hypersensitivity.

Drug Interactions:
Partial agonists (pentazocine, buprenorphine, butorphanol, nalbuphine) may precipitate opioid withdrawal.
Additive CNS depression with alcohol, antihistamines, barbiturates, benzodiazepines, sedatives/hypnotics, antidepressants, antipsychotics, and general anesthetics.
Severe reactions in patients treated with MAO inhibitors.

Monitor: Pain relief, respirations, blood pressure.

PENICILLIN G OR V (Pfizerpen, Pentids; Pen Vee K, V-Cillin K, Ledercillin K, Penapar VK, Uticillin VK, Veetids, Robicillin VK; procaine: Wycillin, Crysticillin; benzathine: Bicillin LA, Permapen)

Pharmacologic Class: Penicillin antibiotic.

Mechanism of Action: Bactericidal effect due to inhibition of synthesis of cell-wall mucopeptide.

Indications:
Infections caused by susceptible organisms: *Streptococcus pneumoniae*, beta-hemolytic streptococci, *Corynebacterium, Bacillus anthracis, Listeria, Neisseria gonorrhoeae*, syphilis.
Prevention of bacterial endocarditis.

Pharmacodynamics:

	Peak	Duration
Oral G,V	0.5–1 hr	4–6 hr, 6–8 hr
IV (pen G)	rapid	3–6 hr
IM (pen G, proc, benz)	15–30 min, 1–4 hr, 12–24 hr	3–6 hr, 1–2 d, 1–4 wk

Route of Excretion: Primarily excreted unchanged by the kidneys.

Dosage:
Oral
  Pen G: Adult: 400,000–600,000 q 4–6 hr.
       Pediatric: <12 yr, 25,000–90,000 units/kg/d in 3–6 divided doses.
  Pen V: Adult: 125–500 mg q 6–8 hr.
       Pediatric: <12 yr, see Pen G.
IM
  Procaine pen: 2.4–4.8 million units with probenecid.
  Benzathine pen: Adult: 1.2–3.0 million units.
              Pediatric: 50,000 u/kg or 300,000–900,000 units.
IV
  Pen G: Adult: 1–30 million units/day.
       Pediatric: 50,000–100,000 u/kg/d in 2–4 divided doses.
Decrease dose with severe renal disease.

Adverse Reactions: Rash, allergic reactions, anaphylaxis, fever; pseudomembranous colitis; interstitial nephritis, hyperkalemia, sodium load; leukopenia, hemolytic anemia; seizures; oral—GI upset; IV—phlebitis; pain at IM site.

Precautions: Use cautiously in patients with renal disease.

Contraindications: Hypersensitivity. May have cross-sensitivity with cephalosporins.

Drug Interactions:
Probenecid blocks penicillin secretion and increases penicillin blood levels.

Activity of penicillins may be diminished when used concomitantly with bacteriostatic antibiotics (e.g., tetracycline).

Do not admix penicillin with aminoglycosides in IV bottle.

Monitor: Temperature, WBC, culture and sensitivity.

PHENOBARBITAL (Luminal)
(Other similar agents: mephobarbital, metharbital)

Pharmacologic Class: Long-acting barbiturate.

Mechanism of Action: Interference with cortical transmission resulting in raised seizure threshold and sedation.

Indications:
Anticonvulsant.
Sedative-hypnotic.
Preoperative anesthetic.

Route of Excretion: Liver (75%), kidneys (25%).

Dosage:
Prevention of seizures (po/IV)
  Adult: 100–300 mg in 2–3 divided doses.
  Pediatric: 4–6 mg/kg/d.
Status epilepticus (IV)
  Adult and children: 10–20 mg/kg, may repeat q 30 min prn, administer at 30–50 mg/min.
Sedative (po, IM)
  Adult: 30–120 mg in 2–3 divided doses.
  Pediatric: 1–3 mg/kg in 3 divided doses.
Hypnotic (po/IM/SC/IV)
  Adult: 100–325 mg hs.
  Pediatric: 3–5 mg/kg hs.

Adverse Reactions: Sedation, confusion, lethargy, dizziness, paradoxical excitation; bradycardia, hypotension (IV); nausea, vomiting, diarrhea, constipation, abdominal pain; rash, fever; megaloblastic anemia, blood dyscrasias; osteomalacia; tolerance, psychological and physical dependence.

Precautions:
Use cautiously in elderly and in patients with hepatic or renal disease.
Abrupt withdrawal may precipitate status asthmaticus.
Warn patients about sedation when driving and operating hazardous machinery.

Contraindications: Patients with respiratory depression, severe pain, prophyria; hypersensitivity, pregnancy, lactation.

Drug Interactions:
Increased metabolism (decreased effect) of oral anticoagulants, oral contraceptives, tricyclics, beta blockers (propranolol, metoprolol), chloramphenicol, corticosteroids, cyclosporine, chlorpromazine, alcohol, acetaminophen, doxycycline.
Increased metabolism with increased toxic metabolite accumulation of meperidine and methoxyflurane.
May increase or decrease levels of phenytoin.
Possible decreased metabolism of barbiturates by propoxyphene,

MAO inhibitors, alcohol.
Possible increased metabolism of barbiturates by alcohol.
Additive CNS depression with alcohol, antihistamines, benzodiazepines, narcotics, antidepressants, and antipsychotics.

Monitor: Phenobarbital level (therapeutic 10–15 mcg/ml), seizure control.

PHENYTOIN (Dilantin)

Pharmacologic Class: Hydantoin anticonvulsant; antiarrhythmic.

Mechanism of Action: Promotes sodium efflux from neurons in motor cortex to prevent spread of seizure activity.

Indications:
Anticonvulsant.
Antiarrhythmic.

Route of Excretion: Metabolized by the liver by zero-order kinetics, half-life increases with increasing dosage.

Dosage:
Anticonvulsant
  Adult: loading dose 10–15 mg/kg, 300–600 mg daily.
  Children: loading dose 5 mg/kg, 4–8 mg/kg/d in 2–3 divided doses.
  Newborns and infants <3 mo: loading dose 15–20 mg/kg, 3–5 mg/kg/d in 3 divided doses.
Status epilepticus
  Adult: 150–250 mg IV, then 100–150 mg 30 minutes later prn.
  Children: 10–15 mg/kg.
Antiarrhythmic
100 mg IV q 5 min or 200–400 mg in 2–4 divided doses.
Altered doses for preterm neonates and elderly.

Adverse Reactions: Nystagmus, ataxia, dizziness, slurred speech, drowsiness, **diplopia,** headache, tremor, lethargy, seizures, coma; hypotension, arrhythmias; **nausea,** hepatitis; interstitial nephritis; hypocalcemia, osteomalacia, hyperglycemia; **gingival hyperplasia,** hirsutism; **rash,** lymphadenopathy; megaloblastic anemia, blood dyscrasias.

Precautions:
Do not administer IV at a rate >50 mg/min.
Use cautiously in elderly, pregnancy, and patients with liver disease, acute intermittent porphyria.

Contraindications: Hypersensitivity, bradycardia, SA block, advanced AV block Adams-Stokes syndrome.

Drug Interactions:
Phenytoin may increase the metabolism of lidocaine, digitoxin, cyclosporine, quinidine, dicumarol, corticosteroids, methadone, disopyramide, metyrapone, theophylline, doxycycline, oral contraceptives.
Possible decreased metabolism of phenytoin by isoniazid, chloramphenicol, cimetidine, disulfiram, phenobarbital (variable effect), phenylbutazone, dicumarol, phenprocoumon, sulfamethizole.
Possible increased metabolism of phenytoin by diazoxide, folic acid, phenobarbital (variable effect), alcohol.
Tricyclics and phenothiazines may lower seizure threshold.
Phenytoin interferes with the effect of levodopa.

Folic acid may decrease the anticonvulsant effect of phenytoin. Increased risk of osteomalacia with acetazolamide.

Monitor: Plasma phenytoin (10–20 mcg/ml), CBC.

POTASSIUM CHLORIDE (Micro K, Klotrix, Klorvess, Kaon Cl, K-Lor, K Tab, Slow K)

Pharmacologic Class: Electrolyte.

Mechanism of Action: Replacement therapy of major intracellular cation.

Indication: Prevention and treatment of potassium deficiency.

Route of Excretion: Renal elimination.

Dosage:
IV for NPO patient: 40–60 mEq/day.
If K >2.5 mEq/L: ≯10 mEq/hr, ≯40 mEq/L, ≯200 mEq/d.
If K <2.5 mEq/L: ≯40 mEq/hr, ≯80 mEq/L, ≯400 mEq/d.
po: prevention, 16–24 mEq/d; treatment, 40–100 mEq/d.

Adverse Reactions: Nausea, vomiting, diarrhea, GI irritation, ulceration; hyperkalemia; arrhythmia; phlebitis.

Precautions:
Use cautiously in elderly, patients with renal disease, cardiac disease.
Avoid wax matrix tablets in patients with impaired GI motility or enlarged left atria.
Monitor acid-base balance before determining treatment plan.

Contraindications: Hyperkalemia, severe renal disease, untreated Addison's disease, patients treated with potassium-sparing diuretics.

Drug Interactions:
Increased risk of hyperkalemia in patients treated with amiloride, triamterene, spironolactone, captopril, enalapril.
Anticholinergic preparations may increase risk of GI ulceration from solid oral KCl due to slowed motility.

Monitor: Potassium, acid-base status, chloride; ECG.

PRAZOSIN (Minipress)

Pharmacologic Class: α_1-adrenoceptor antagonist antihypertensive.

Mechanism of Action: Blockade of postsynaptic alpha-adrenergic receptors resulting in dilation of arterioles and veins. Results in lower blood pressure and increased cardiac output without reflex tachycardia.

Indications:
Hypertension.
CHF.

Route of Excretion: Primarily hepatically metabolized but metabolites are active.

Dosage: 2–40 mg/d in 2–3 divided doses.

Adverse Reactions: Dizziness, headache, drowsiness, lethargy, nervousness, depression, paresthesias; **hypotension, palpitations,** edema, syncope, tachycardia, angina; nausea, vomiting, diarrhea, abdominal pain; impotence, urinary frequency; blurred vision, dry mouth.

Precautions:
Syncopal effect may occur with first dose; give at bedtime.
Use cautiously in patients with renal disease.

Contraindications: Hypersensitivity.

Drug Interactions: Enhanced "first-dose" syncopal effect in patients treated with beta blockers.

Monitor: Blood pressure, heart rate.

PREDNISONE (Meticorten, Deltasone, Orasone)

Pharmacologic Class: Glucocorticoid—intermediate acting.

Mechanism of Action: Anti-inflammatory action and immunosuppressant effect due to a variety of effects: inhibition of protein synthesis, inhibition of prostaglandin synthesis, impaired cell-mediated immunity by reduction in T lymphocytes, decreased neutrophil migration, decreased capillary permeability, vasoconstriction.

Indications:
Used for autoimmune, allergic, and inflammatory disorders, malignancies.
Immunosuppression following transplantation.

Route of Excretion: Hepatically metabolized with plasma half-life 60 min; biologic $t^1/_2$ 18–36 hr.

Dosage:
Oral—5 mg prednisone equivalent to 25 mg cortisone, 0.75 mg dexamethasone.
Adult: 5–200 mg/d in 1–4 divided doses.
Pediatric: 0.1–2.0 mg/kg/d in 4 divided doses.

Adverse Reactions: Adrenal suppression, depression, stunted growth in children, euphoria, insomnia, psychoses; **acne,** hyperpigmentation, hirsutism, **petechiae, ecchymoses, impaired wound healing,** moon facies, buffalo hump; glaucoma, cataracts; weight gain, nausea, vomiting, peptic ulceration, pancreatitis; azotemia, edema, sodium and water retention, hypokalemia, **hyperglycemia,** amenorrhea, thromboembolism, myopathy, osteoporosis, infections.

Precautions:
Chronic use leads to adrenal suppression; patients will require supplemental doses during stress. Do not discontinue abruptly.
May mask signs of infections; may reactivate latent TB; may exacerbate fungal infections.
Monitor glucose carefully in patients with diabetes mellitus or latent DM.

Contraindications: Systemic fungal infections, administration of live virus vaccines.

Drug Interactions:
Phenobarbital, phenytoin, and rifampin increase metabolism and may decrease effect of prednisone.
Oral contraceptives (estrogens), isoniazid, and troleandomycin may inhibit steroid metabolism.
Increased requirement for insulin and oral hypoglycemics in diabetics.
Enhanced metabolism of isoniazid and salicylates.
Inhibition of coumarin response by steroids.
Increased risk of hypokalemia with potassium-wasting diuretics, and amphotericin B.

Monitor: WBC with differential, weight, edema, blood pressure, potassium, glucose.

PROBENECID (Benemid)

Pharmacologic Class: Uricosuric agent.

Mechanism of Action: Inhibition of renal tubular reabsorption of urate, thus increasing urinary urate excretion and decreasing serum uric acid levels.

Indications:
Treatment of hyperuricemia.
Decrease penicillin renal excretion, causing increased and prolonged penicillin levels.

Route of Excretion: Metabolized in the liver to active metabolites which are renally excreted.

Dosage:
Hyperuricemia: Start at 250 mg bid × 1 week, then increase by 500 mg daily. May continue to increase every 4 weeks until maximum dose 2000 mg/d in 2 divided doses.
With penicillin or cephalosporin:
  Adult: 500 mg qid.
  Pediatric: (>2 yr) start 25 mg/kg, raise to 10 mg/kg qid.
Treatment of gonorrhea: Give 1 g ½ hour before penicillin or amoxicillin.

Adverse Reactions: Headache, dizziness; anorexia, **nausea**, vomiting, **diarrhea**, hepatitis; sore gums, flushing, rash, allergic reactions; aplastic anemia, hemolytic anemia (G-6 PD deficiency); urinary frequency, urate nephrolithiasis; exacerbation of gout.

Precautions:
Probenecid is probably ineffective with GFR < 30 ml/min.
Increase fluid intake and alkalinize urine to decrease risk of renal colic from urate stones.
Use cautiously in patients with G-6-PD deficiency, acute intermittent porphyria, and history of peptic ulcer disease.

Contraindications: Hypersensitivity.

Drug Interactions:
Probenecid decreases the renal excretion of penicillins, cephalosporins, dapsone, dyphylline, aminosalicylic acid, methotrexate, sulfinpyrazone, sulfonamides, indomethacin, naproxen, chlorpropamide.
Salicylates and pyrazinamide antagonize uricosuric action of probenecid.

Monitor: Serum uric acid, frequency of gouty attacks, and urate-induced renal colic.

PROCAINAMIDE (Pronestyl, Promine, Procan SR, Pronestyl SR)

Pharmacologic Class: Type 1 antiarrhythmic.

Mechanism of Action: Depresses myocardial excitability with slowed conduction in the atrium, His bundle, and ventricle.

Indications: Atrial and ventricular arrhythmias.

Route of Excretion: Partially metabolized in the liver to N-acetyl procainamide (NAPA), an active metabolite. NAPA and 40–70% of drug excreted unchanged renally; half-life: procainamide, 2.5–4.5 hr; NAPA 6–7 hr.

Dosage:
Oral:
   Initial 12 mg/kg, then 6 mg/kg q 3 hr; sustained release 12 mg/kg q 6 hr.
IM: 500–1000 mg q 4–8 hr.
IV bolus: 100 mg q 5 min, maximum total 1000 mg.
IV infusion: 500 mg initial, then 2–6 mg/min.
Reduced dose in patients with renal or hepatic insufficiency, CHF.

Adverse Reactions: Weakness, confusion, psychosis, seizures; hypotension (IV), ventricular arrhythmias; anorexia, nausea, vomiting, diarrhea, dysgeusia, acute hepatitis; blood dyscrasias (leukopenia); systemic lupus erythematosus syndrome; fever, chills, rash, allergic reaction.

Precautions:
Administer IV bolus procainamide at a rate not faster than 20–50 mg/min.
Use cautiously in patients with severe digitalis intoxication, second- and third-degree heart block, bundle branch block, myocardial infarction.

Contraindicated: Myasthenia gravis, complete AV block.

Drug Interactions:
Cimetidine decreases renal excretion of procainamide and NAPA.
Procainamide may antagonize the effect of cholinergic drugs.
Increased hypotensive effect with antihypertensives.
Enhanced effect with neuromuscular blocking agents.
Enhanced anticholinergic effect.
Additive toxicity with other antiarrhythmics.

Monitor: ECG, procainamide level (therapeutic 4–10 mcg/ml), combined procainamide and NAPA < 30 mcg/ml, ANA, WBC.

PROCHLORPERAZINE (Compazine)

Pharmacologic Class: Piperazine phenothiazine, antiemetic.

Mechanism of Action: Blocks dopamine 2 receptors in the brain.

Indications: Prevention and treatment of nausea and vomiting.

Route of Excretion: Metabolized by the liver.

Dosage:

	po	Rectal	IM
Adult	5–10 mg tid–qid; spansule 10 mg q 12 hr	25 mg bid	5–10 mg q 3–4 hr prn; maximum 40 mg/d
Children (>2yr)	2.5 mg 1–3 times/d	Same as oral	0.132 mg/kg × 1

Adverse Reactions: Sedation, depression, extrapyramidal reactions, seizures, tardive dyskinesia; orthostatic hypotension, tachycardia, CHF, arrhythmias; urticaria, rash, photosensitivity, skin pigmentation; impotence, gynecomastia, amenorrhea, galactorrhea; dry mouth, weight gain, constipation, cholestatic jaundice; urinary retention; blurred vision; blood dyscrasias (leukopenia).

Precautions:
Use cautiously in elderly and in patients with prostatic hypertrophy, seizure disorder, glaucoma.
Caution patients about sedation concerning driving and operating hazardous machinery.

Contraindications: Hypersensitivity (cross-sensitivity with other phenothiazines may occur), coma, severe depression, Parkinson's disease, blood dyscrasias, severe liver or cardiac disease.

Drug Interactions:
Decreased absorption of phenothiazines by antacids, anticholinergics.
Phenothiazines may inhibit metabolism of tricyclics, phenytoin, propranolol.
Phenothiazines may inhibit effect of levodopa, guanethidine, amphetamine.
May increase effect of antihypertensives, CNS depressants, and anticholinergics.

Monitor: Symptomatic response, WBC, LFTs, extrapyramidal reactions.

PROPRANOLOL (Inderal)

Pharmacologic Class: β-adrenoceptor antagonist, antihypertensive.

Mechanism of Action: Inhibition of beta 1 and beta 2 receptors, resulting in decreased blood pressure, heart rate, and cardiac output.

Indications:
Hypertension.
Angina pectoris.
Tachyarrhythmias.
Post MI to decrease mortality and risk of reinfarction.
Adjunct with alpha blocker for pheochromocytoma.
Prophylaxis of migraine.
Symptoms of idiopathic hypertrophic subaortic stenosis (IHSS).

Route of Excretion: Lipophilic agent which crosses blood-brain barrier and is hepatically metabolized.

Dosage:
HT: 80–240 mg/d in 2–3 divided doses, once daily for sustained release (SR).
Angina: 30–320 mg/d in 3–4 divided doses.
Arrhythmias: 30–120 mg/d in 3–4 divided doses.
Post MI: 180–240 mg/d in 2–4 divided doses.
Pheochromocytoma: 30–60 mg/d in 2–4 divided doses.
Migraine prophylaxis: 80–240 mg/d in 2–4 divided doses or once daily for SR.
IHSS: 60–160 mg/d in 3–4 divided doses or once daily for SR.

Adverse Reactions: Drowsiness, weakness, fatigue, depression, insomnia, lightheadedness; blurred vision; **bradycardia**, hypotension, CHF; bronchoconstriction, cough, rhinitis; nausea, vomiting, diarrhea; impotence; Raynaud's phenomenon, SLE syndrome.

Precautions:
Abrupt withdrawal may precipitate MI, angina, or arrhythmias.
Use cautiously in diabetics—may mask symptoms of hypoglycemia and prolong recovery.
May mask symptoms of thyrotoxicosis.
Use cautiously in patients with impaired hepatic function, Wolff-Parkinson-White syndrome, and patients treated with MAO inhibitors.

Contraindications: Uncompensated CHF, bradycardia, asthma, COPD, pregnancy, lactation.

Drug Interactions:
Increased clearance of propranolol by barbiturates and rifampin.
Decreased clearance of propranolol by cimetidine and chlorpromazine.
Propranolol may decrease the clearance of lidocaine, chlorpromazine, and theophylline.

- Exaggerated response (hypertension and/or bradycardia) in patients treated with methyldopa, epinephrine, phenylephrine, phenylpropanolamine, or upon abrupt withdrawal of clonidine.
- Smoking reduces effect of propranolol on angina.
- Additive hypotension with phenothiazines, antihypertensives, prazosin (postural hypotension), nitrates, and halothane.
- Enhanced cardiac depressant effect with nifedipine and verapamil.
- Propranolol may antagonize the effect of isoproterenol, theophylline, or beta stimulants.
- Indomethacin may decrease the effect of propranolol.

Monitor: Blood pressure, heart rate.

QUINIDINE (Q. sulfate: Cin Quin, Quinora, Quinidex; Q. gluconate: Duraquin, Quinaglute; Q. polygalacturonate: Cardioquin)

Pharmacologic Class: Type I antiarrhythmic.

Mechanism of Action: Sodium channel depressor, depresses myocardial excitability and conduction.

Indications: Arrhythmias—atrial and ventricular.

Route of Excretion: Liver (60–80%), kidneys (10–30%); half-life 6–7 hours.

Pharmacodynamics:

	% Quinidine	Peak	Duration
Q. sulfate	83%	0.5–1.5 hr	6–8 hr
Q. sulfate (S.R.)	83%	4 hr	8–12 hr
Q. gluconate (S.R.)	62%	3–4 hr	6–8 hr
Q. polygalacturonate	60%	6 hr	8–12 hr
IM		0.5–1.5 hr	6–8 hr
IV		Immediate	6–8 hr

Dosage:
Oral
　Q. sulfate: 200–400 mg q 5–8 hr; SR 300–600 mg q 8–12 hr.
　Q. gluconate: 324–648 mg q 8–12 hr.
　Q. polygalacturonate: 275 mg q 8–12 hr.
IM: 600 mg initial, then 400 mg q 2 hr prn.
IV: 330–750 mg, infuse slowly at 16 mg/min.

Adverse Reactions: Headache, vertigo, tinnitus; blurred vision; widened QRS, arrhythmia, syncope, heart block, hypotension; **nausea,** vomiting, **diarrhea, abdominal pain,** hepatitis; hemolytic anemia, thrombocytopenia, leukopenia; SLE syndrome; rash, pruritus, fever.

Precautions:
Digitalize patient before using quinidine in atrial flutter.
Reduced doses in elderly, CHF, hepatic dysfunction.
Administer test dose to determine if patient has idiosyncratic reaction.
Maintain normal potassium balance in quinidine-treated patients.

Contraindications: AV conduction defects, digitalis intoxication, renal tubular acidosis, hypersensitivity, or idiosyncratic reaction to quinidine.

Drug Interactions:
Increased digoxin concentration due to decreased clearance.
Decrease renal excretion of quinidine by sodium bicarbonate, acetazolamide, and magnesium-aluminum hydroxide.

Enhanced metabolism of quinidine by rifampin, phenytoin, and phenobarbital.

Decreased metabolism of quinidine by cimetidine.

Addition of amiodarone may cause arrhythmias and increased quinidine level.

May antagonize the effect of cholinergic drugs. Additive hypoprothrombinemic effect with oral anticoagulants.

May rarely cause excessive paralysis when used with pancuronium, curare.

Monitor: ECG (QRS duration), heart rate, blood pressure, quinidine level (therapeutic 3–6 mcg/ml), CBC.

RANITIDINE (Zantac)

Pharmacologic Class: H_2-receptor antagonist.

Mechanism of Action: Inhibits histamine-stimulated gastric acid secretion.

Indications:
Prophylaxis and treatment of duodenal ulcers.
Treatment of active, benign gastric ulcers.
Zollinger-Ellison syndrome.

Route of Excretion: Oral: hepatic, 70%; renal, 30%; parenteral: renal, 70–80%; hepatic, 20–30%.

Dosage:
Oral: 150 mg bid.
IM/IV soluset (over 5–20 min): 50 mg q 6–8 hr.
Reduce dose with Cr Cl < 50 ml/min.

Adverse Reactions: Headache, malaise, dizziness; arrhythmias; nausea, vomiting, abdominal pain, constipation, hepatitis; rash, allergic reactions.

Precautions: Use cautiously in elderly and in patients with renal and hepatic disease.

Contraindications: Hypersensitivity.

Drug Interactions:
Antacids may decrease ranitidine's GI absorption.
Smoking reduces effect of ranitidine.

Monitor: Symptomatic response, stool guaiac, repeat radiographic studies, or endoscopy.

RIFAMPIN (Rifadin, Rimactane)

Pharmacologic Class: Antitubercular agent.

Mechanism of Action: Inhibits RNA synthesis in bacteria by forming a complex with DNA-dependent RNA polymerase.

Indications:
In combination with other antitubercular drugs for treatment of tuberculosis.
Asymptomatic carrier of *Neisseria meningitidis*.
In synergy with other antibiotics for staphylococcal infections.

Route of Excretion: Primarily metabolized by the liver and excreted through biliary tract; $t^{1/2}$ 3 hr.

Dosage:
Adult: 600 mg/d.
Children: 10–20 mg/kg/d.
Treatment for 4 days for meningococcal carriers.
Administer on empty stomach.

Adverse Reactions: Headache, drowsiness, fatigue, confusion; anorexia, **nausea**, vomiting, **diarrhea, abdominal pain**; myalgias, arthralgias; rashes; blood dyscrasias, hemolytic anemia; acute interstitial nephritis; flulike syndrome; menstrual irregularities, osteomalacia.

Precautions: Use cautiously in patients with liver disease or other hepatotoxic drugs.
Do not use for intermittent therapy.
Red-orange discoloration of body fluids.

Contraindications: Hypersensitivity; pregnancy and lactation.

Drug Interactions:
Rifampin may increase metabolism of warfarin, quinidine, disopyramide, cyclosporine, metoprolol, propranolol, isoniazid, oral contraceptives, corticosteroids, digitoxin, methadone, clofibrate, tolbutamide, chlorpropamide, diazepam, halazepam, clorazepate, prazepam.
Aminosalicylic acid (PAS) may decrease GI absorption of rifampin.
Potential increased hepatotoxicity with halothane and isoniazid.

Monitor: CBC, LFTs.

SODIUM BICARBONATE

Pharmacologic Class: Alkalinizing agent, systemic antacid.

Mechanism of Action: Increases bicarbonate, buffers excess hydrogen ion, raises pH.

Indications:
Metabolic acidosis.
Urinary alkalinization.
Antacid (oral).

Route of Excretion: Renally eliminated.

Dosage:
IV
   Adult: (7.5–8.4%) 1 mEq/kg, then 0.5 mEq/kg q 10 minutes or calculate deficit = (0.5) (wt kg) (desired − actual HCO_3).
   Child: (4.2%) 1–2 mEq/kg then 1 mEq/kg q 10 minutes or calculate deficit = (0.3) (wt kg) (desired − actual HCO_3).
Oral: 0.5–3.0 mEq/kg/d in 2–3 divided doses; higher doses may be needed for urinary alkalinization and treatment of renal tubular acidosis.

Side Effects: Pulmonary edema, hypertension; **metabolic alkalosis, hypernatremia, edema, sodium and water retention;** hypocalcemic tetany; gastric distention, belching, flatulence (oral only); phlebitis (IV).

Precautions:
Use cautiously in patients with CHF and renal failure and with those treated with glucocorticoids due to sodium load.
Use cautiously in hypocalcemic patients; sodium bicarbonate may precipitate tetany.

Contraindications: Metabolic or respiratory alkalosis.

Drug Interactions:
Decreased renal clearance of amphetamines, ephedrine, pseudophedrine, quinidine.
Increased renal clearance of lithium carbonate, salicylates, barbiturates, tetracyclines (doxycycline).
Sodium bicarbonate decreases the effectiveness of methenamine.
Parenteral solutions with sodium bicarbonate and calcium may cause precipitation of calcium complexes.
Oral therapy with sodium bicarbonate and calcium salts may lead to milk alkali syndrome.

Monitor: Serum bicarbonate or CO_2 content, ABG, urinary pH.

SODIUM POLYSTYRENE SULFONATE (Kayexalate, SPS)

Pharmacologic Class: Potassium exchange resin.

Mechanism of Action: Exchanges sodium for potassium ions in the large intestine, resulting in enhanced excretion of potassium in the stool.

Indications: Prevention and treatment of hyperkalemia.

Route of Excretion: Fecal.

Dosage:
Oral: 15–25 g 1–4 times daily in water or sorbitol suspension.
Rectal enema: 30–50 g q 4–6 hr.

Adverse Reactions: Anorexia, nausea, vomiting, constipation, fecal impaction; hypokalemia, hypocalcemia, sodium retention.

Precautions:
Frequently administered with sorbitol to prevent constipation and fecal impaction.
Use cautiously in elderly and in patients with severe cardiac disease.
For severe hyperkalemia, use more rapidly acting treatments (IV calcium, sodium bicarbonate, and glucose with insulin).

Drug Interactions: Systemic alkalosis may occur in patients treated with SPS and magnesium- or calcium-containing antacids.

Monitor: Serum potassium.

SPIRONOLACTONE (Aldactone)

Pharmacologic Class: Potassium-sparing diuretic.

Mechanism of Action: Competitive inhibitor of aldosterone, which causes excretion of sodium and water, conservation of potassium and hydrogen.

Indications:
Primary hyperaldosteronism.
Edema associated with cirrhosis.
In conjunction with other agents for the treatment of hypertension, edema associated with nephrotic syndrome, CHF.
Prevention of hypokalemia.
Hirsutism.

Route of Excretion: Metabolized in the liver to active metabolite, canrenone.

Dosage:
Adult: 25–400 mg/day.
Pediatric: 3.3 mg/kg/d.

Adverse Reactions: Drowsiness, headache, ataxia; **anorexia, nausea,** vomiting, **diarrhea,** abdominal cramps; **hyperkalemia,** hyperchloremic metabolic acidosis; gynecomastia, impotence, menstrual irregularities, hirsutism; rash, urticaria; association with breast cancer.

Precautions:
Use cautiously in elderly.
Maximum effect of each dosage adjustment may take 3–5 days; do not increase dose too rapidly.
Avoid concomitant administration of KCl, other potassium-sparing diuretics and salt substitutes.

Contraindications: Renal failure, hyperkalemia, pregnancy, lactation, hypersensitivity.

Drug Interactions:
Increased risk of hyperkalemia with KCl, salt substitutes, triamterene, amiloride, captopril, enalapril, lisinopril.
May decrease renal excretion of lithium.
Salicylates may antagonize natriuretic effect of spironolactone.
Spironolactone may decrease renal excretion of digoxin, increase metabolism of digitoxin, and produce false elevations in some digoxin serum assays.

Monitor: Potassium, weight, intake and output, blood pressure.

SUCRALFATE (Carafate)

Pharmacologic Class: Mucosal barrier agent.

Mechanism of Action: An aluminum-sucrose complex which locally forms a proteinaceous complex at ulcer site and inhibits pepsin activity.

Indications:
Treatment of duodenal ulcers.
Treatment of gastric ulcers.
Reflex esophagitis.
Hyperphosphatemia.

Route of Excretion: Fecal.

Dosage: 1 g qid (1 hr ac + hs).

Adverse Reactions: Dizziness, drowsiness, vertigo; dry mouth, nausea, indigestion, **constipation,** diarrhea; rash, pruritus; hypophosphatemia.

Precautions: Ulcer disease may recur.

Contraindications: Hypersensitivity.

Drug Interactions:
May decrease GI absorption of cimetidine, phenytoin, tetracycline, or warfarin. Cannot be administered with H_2-receptor antagonists or antacids (needs acid pH).

Monitor: Healing of ulcer by endoscopy or radiographic examination, stool guaiac.

SULFASALAZINE (Azulfidine, SAS, Azaline)

Pharmacologic Class: Sulfonamide.

Mechanism of Action: Sulfasalazine is split in the colon into sulfapyridine (antibacterial agent) and 5-amino salicylic acid (5 ASA, anti-inflammatory agent).

Indications:
Ulcerative colitis.
Rheumatoid arthritis.
Crohn's disease.

Route of Excretion: 5 ASA primarily excreted in feces; sulfapyridine mostly renally eliminated.

Dosage:
Adults: 1–8g/d in 3–4 divided doses.
Children: 30–60 mg/kg/d in 3–6 divided doses.

Adverse Reactions: Headache, drowsiness, vertigo, tinnitus, ataxia, depression, seizures, peripheral neuropathy; **anorexia, nausea, vomiting, diarrhea,** abdominal pains, hepatitis, pancreatitis; crystalluria; blood dyscrasias, hemolytic anemia (G-6 PD deficiency); infertility; rash, fever, urticaria, photosensitivity, allergic reactions; skin and urine discoloration (orange-yellow).

Precautions: Use cautiously in patients with impaired hepatic or renal function.

Contraindications: Hypersensitivity (salicylates or sulfonamides), porphyria, children < 2 yr, pregnancy, lactation, G-6-PD deficiency, patients with intestinal or urinary obstruction.

Drug Interactions:
May decrease absorption of ferrous sulfate, folic acid, and digoxin.
 May increase hypoprothrombinemic effect of oral anticoagulants.

Monitor: CBC.

SULFISOXAZOLE (Gantrisin, Gulfusin, SK-Soxazole)

Pharmacologic Class: Sulfonamide antibiotic.

Mechanism of Action: Blocks para-aminobenzoic acid (PABA) and inhibits folic acid synthesis.

Indications:
Infections caused by susceptible organisms: *E. coli, Proteus mirabilis, H. influenzae, Nocardia.*
Used in combination therapy for *Toxoplasma gonadii*, and *P. falciparum.*

Route of Excretion: Primarily excreted in urine.

Dosage:

	Adult	Children
Oral	4–8g/d in 4–6 divided doses	150 mg/kg/d in 4–6 divided doses
IM	100 mg/kg/d in 2–3 divided doses	Same as adult
SC	100 mg/kg/d in 3 divided doses	Same as adult
IV	100 mg/kg in 4 divided doses	Same as adult

Adverse Reactions: Headache, drowsiness, vertigo, tinnitus, ataxia, depression, seizures, peripheral neuropathy; **anorexia, nausea, vomiting,** diarrhea, abdominal pains, hepatitis, pancreatitis; crystalluria, blood dyscrasias, hemolytic anemia (G-6-PD deficiency); rash, fever, urticaria, photosensitivity, allergic reactions.

Precautions: Use cautiously in patients with impaired hepatic or renal function.

Contraindications: Hypersensitivity to sulfonamides, porphyria, children < 2 mo, pregnancy, lactation, G-6-PD deficiency.

Drug Interactions:
May require decreased doses of thiopental and methotrexate due to competition for protein binding.
Local anesthetics and PABA may antagonize the effect of sulfonamides.
May enhance the effect of oral hypoglycemic and oral anticoagulants.

Monitor: Temperature, WBC, culture and sensitivity.

TAMOXIFEN (Nolvadex)

Pharmacologic Class: Antiestrogen antineoplastic.

Mechanism of Action: Competes with estradiol for estrogen-binding receptors in breast tissue.

Indications: Breast cancer in postmenopausal women.

Route of Excretion: Metabolized by the liver, undergoes enterohepatic recirculation, fecal excretion; half-life >7 days.

Dosage: 10–20 mg po bid.

Adverse Reactions: Dizziness, headache, depression, blurred vision, cataracts; **nausea, vomiting;** edema, hypercalcemia; thromboembolism, blood dyscrasias; vaginal bleeding, vaginal discharge; rash, **hot flashes;** bone and tumor pain.

Precautions:
Use cautiously in patients with leukopenia or thrombocytopenia.
Avoid in pregnancy, lactation.

Contraindications: Hypersensitivity.

Drug Interactions:
Decrease effectiveness of estrogens.
Increases effectiveness of MPA in treatment of endometrial carcinoma.

Monitor: Calcium, CBC, tumor response.

TERBUTALINE (Brethaire, Brethine, Bricanyl)

Pharmacologic Class: β_2-adrenoceptor stimulant.

Mechanism of Action: Beta 2 agonists stimulate adenyl cyclase, causing increased cyclic AMP and resulting in bronchodilation.

Indications:
Bronchodilator for asthma or COPD.
Premature labor.

Route of Excretion: Partially hepatically metabolized.

Dosage:
Oral:
  Adult 2.5–5.0 mg tid.
  Pediatric: (12–15 yr) 2.5 mg tid.
Inhalation: 2 inhalations q 4–6 hr.
SC: 0.25 mg may repeat in 15–30 min.

Adverse Reactions: Restlessness, anxiety, tremor, headache, blurred vision, insomnia; **tachycardia,** palpitations, hypertension; nausea, vomiting, heartburn; hyperglycemia; urinary retention; hypokalemia.

Precautions:
Use cautiously in patients with cardiac disease, hyperthyroidism, diabetes, prostatic hypertrophy, seizures, glaucoma.
Not recommended for children <12 yr.
Tolerance and bronchospasm may occur with prolonged and excessive use of inhaled terbutaline.

Contraindications: Hypersensitivity, tachycardia.

Drug Interactions:
Beta blockers may antagonize therapeutic effect.
Severe hypertension in patients treated with MAO inhibitors.
Additive adrenergic effect with tricyclics.

Monitor: Heart rate, blood pressure, symptomatic relief.

TETRACYCLINE (Achromycin, Sumycin, Panmycin, Tetracyn, Polycycline, Cyclopar)
(Other antibiotics with similar spectrum of action: demeclocycline, doxycycline, methacycline, minocycline, oxytetracycline, chlortetracycline)

Pharmacologic Class: Antibiotic.

Mechanism of Action: Inhibition of protein synthesis.

Indications: Infections caused by susceptible organisms: *E. coli*, *Klebsiella*, group A beta-hemolytic streptococci, *H. influenzae*, *Legionella pneumophilia*, *Neisseria*, *Clostridium*, *Listeria monocytogenes*, *Bacillus anthracis*, *Nocardia*, *Proprionibacterium acnes*, *Treponema*, *Chlamydia*, *Mycoplasma*, *Rickettsia*, *Corynebacterium acnes* (severe acne).

Route of Excretion: Primarily renally eliminated, half-life 6–10 hr.

Dosage:
Oral
 Adult: 1000–2000 mg in 2–4 divided doses; maintenance for acne, 125–500 mg/d.
 Children (>8 yr): 25–50 mg/kg in 2–4 divided doses.
IM
 Adult: 300 mg in 1–3 divided doses.
 Children (>8 yr): 15–25 mg/kg in 2–3 divided doses.
IV
 Adult: 500–1000 mg/d in 2 divided doses.
 Children (>8 yr): 10–20 mg/kg/d in 2 divided doses.

Adverse Reactions: Anorexia, nausea, vomiting, diarrhea, esophageal ulcers, black hairy tongue, hepatitis; azotemia; rash, photosensitivity, allergic reaction; superinfection (e.g., staphylococcal enterocolitis, pseudomembranous colitis); blood dyscrasias; phlebitis (IV), pain at IM site.

Precautions: Use cautiously in patients with hepatic or renal disease, or postpartum patients.

Contraindications: Children <8 yr, pregnancy, lactation, hypersensitivity.

Drug Interactions:
Antacids, iron, and dairy products may decrease GI absorption.
Enhanced hypoprothrombinemic effect of oral anticoagulants.
Tetracycline may increase digoxin's bioavailability.
May decrease effect of oral contraceptives.
Concomitant use of tetracycline and diuretics may increase risk of azotemia.
Increased nephrotoxicity with methoxyflurane.

Monitor: Temperature, CBC, culture and sensitivity.

THEOPHYLLINE (Bronkodyl Elixophyllin, Quibron, Phyllin, Theolair, Theobid, TheoDur)
IV Aminophylline (86% theophylline)

Pharmacologic Class: Methylxanthine, bronchodilator, and CNS stimulant.

Mechanism of Action: May work by inhibiting phosphodiesterase, resulting in increased cyclic AMP concentrations and bronchodilation.

Indication: Bronchodilator for the treatment of asthma or COPD.

Route of Excretion: 85–90% metabolized by the liver. Decreased plasma clearance in elderly, neonates, and in patients with CHF or liver disease. Increased clearance in cigarette smokers.

Dosage:
Individualize, maintain serum theophylline conc. = 10–20 mcg/ml.
IV aminophylline
 Adult: loading dose 7.5 mg/kg, maintenance 3.8 mg/kg q 8 hr.
 Pediatric: loading dose 7.5 mg/kg, maintenance 3.8–5.1 mg/kg q 6 hr.
Oral
 Adult: 2–16 mg/kg/day in divided doses (interval depends on preparation, some sustained-release preparations available).
 Pediatric: 12–16 mg/kg/day in 1–4 divided doses.

Adverse Reactions: (Most often at serum concentrations >20 mcg/ml) anorexia, **nausea, vomiting,** diarrhea; **anxiety, nervousness,** insomnia, headache, **seizures, tachycardia, arrhythmias,** hypotension.

Precautions:
Decreased doses in neonates, elderly, patients with CHF or liver disease.
Use with caution in patients with severe cardiovascular disease, severe hypertension, acute myocardial infarction, hyperthyroidism, and peptic ulcer disease.

Contraindications: Hypersensitivity to xanthines, uncontrolled arrhythmias.

Drug Interactions:
Drugs that may increase theophylline concentrations include allopurinol, cimetidine, clindamycin, erythromycin, influenza virus vaccine, lincomycin, rifampin, thiabendazole, troleandomycin.
Drugs that may decrease theophylline concentrations include cigarette and marijuana smoking, carbamazepine, phenobarbital.
Theophylline increases the renal excretion of lithium carbonate.
Beta-adrenergic blocking agents may antagonize effect of theophylline and decrease its clearance.

Monitor: Serum theophylline concentration (normal 10–20 mcg/ml), blood pressure, heart rate.

TRAZODONE (Desyrel)

Pharmacologic Class: Antidepressant.

Mechanism of Action: Unknown, may inhibit serotonin's neuronal uptake.

Indications: Depression.

Route of Excretion: Metabolized by the liver; half-life 5–9 hr.

Dosage: 150–600 mg/d in 3 divided doses.

Adverse Reactions: Drowsiness, dizziness, fatigue, headache, insomnia, impaired memory, confusion, slurred speech, hallucinations, seizures; blurred vision; **hypotension,** tachycardia, palpitations, syncope, hypertension; **dry mouth,** nausea, vomiting, diarrhea, constipation, sialorrhea; urinary frequency, impotence, priapism; blood dyscrasias; myalgias.

Precautions:
Use cautiously in patient with cardiovascular disease—may cause drowsiness. Caution patients concerning driving and operating hazardous machinery.

Contraindications:
Hypersensitivity.
Recent myocardial infarction.
Avoid concurrent electroshock therapy.

Drug Interactions:
May increase digoxin or phenytoin levels.
Additive hypotension with antihypertensives (except clonidine—then hypertension) and nitrates.
Additive CNS depression with alcohol, antihistamines, barbiturates, opioids, and sedatives/hypnotics.

Monitor: Symptomatic response (onset 1–4 weeks), blood pressure, heart rate.

TRIAMTERENE (Dyrenium, in Dyazide and Maxzide)

Pharmacologic Class: Potassium-sparing diuretic.

Mechanism of Action: Acts directly on renal tubule to increase excretion of sodium and water and to decrease secretion of potassium and hydrogen.

Indications:
Frequently used in combination with other diuretics to treat hypertension and edema.
Prevents or treats diuretic-induced hypokalemia.

Pharmacodynamics:

	Onset	Peak	Duration
Oral	2 hr	6–8 hr	12–16 hr

Route of Excretion: Metabolized by the liver to active metabolite, which is renally eliminated.

Dosage: 100–300 mg/d in 2–3 divided doses.

Adverse Reactions: Hyperkalemia, nephrolithiasis, interstitial nephritis; dry mouth, headache; hypotension; **nausea,** vomiting, diarrhea; blood dyscrasias, megaloblastic anemia (in cirrhotics); rash, photosensitivity, allergic reaction.

Precautions: Use cautiously in patients with diabetes, impaired liver function.

Contraindications: Hyperkalemia, renal dysfunction, hypersensitivity.

Drug Interactions:
Increased risk of hyperkalemia with KCl, salt substitutes, spironolactone, amiloride, captopril, enalapril, lisinopril.
May decrease renal excretion of lithium.
Increase in serum digoxin levels.
Increases risk of acute renal failure in patients treated with indomethacin and triamterene.
Additive hypotensive effect with antihypertensives and nitrates.

Monitor: Serum potassium, weight, intake and output, blood pressure.

TRIMETHOPRIM-SULFAMETHOXAZOLE
(Co-Trimoxazole, TMP-SMZ, Septra, Bactrim)

Pharmacologic Class: Antibiotic.

Mechanism of Action: Interferes with folic acid synthesis.

Indications: Infections caused by susceptible organisms: *E. coli, Klebsiella, Enterobacter, Proteus, Shigella, Salmonella, Serratia, Pseudomonas pseudomallei, H. influenzae, Streptococcus pneumoniae,* group A beta-hemolytic streptococci, *Pneumocystis; Nocardia, Gonococcus.*

Route of Excretion: SMZ primarily metabolized by the liver to inactive metabolites; TMP primarily renally excreted; half-life TMP 8–11 hr, SMZ 7–12 hr.

Dosage:
Oral
  Adult: 160 mg TMP/800 mg SMZ q 12 hr.
  Pediatric: 4 mg/kg TMP/20 mg/kg SMZ q 12 hr.
IV: 8 mg/kg TMP/40 mg/kg SMZ daily in 2–4 divided doses.
Pneumocystis carinii pneumonitis:
Oral (adult and children): 20 mg/kg TMP/100 mg/kg SMZ daily in 4 divided doses.
IV: 15–20 mg/kg TMP/75–100 mg/kg SMZ daily in 3–4 divided doses.
Reduced doses with Cr Cl < 30 ml/minute.

Adverse Reactions: Nausea, vomiting, diarrhea, glossitis, stomatitis, hepatitis, pancreatitis, pseudomembranous colitis; crystalluria; blood dyscrasias, hemolytic anemia (G-6-PD deficiency), megaloblastic anemia; fever, rash, pruritus, allergic reaction; phlebitis (IV).

Precautions:
Trimethoprim may impair tubular secretion of creatinine and raise serum creatinine, without affecting GFR.
Use cautiously in patients with impaired renal or hepatic disease, folate deficiency, asthma.

Contraindications: Megaloblastic anemia, G-6-PD deficiency, porphyria, hypersensitivity to trimethoprim or sulfonamides.

Drug Interactions:
Additive hypoprothrombinemic effect with warfarin.
May decrease hepatic clearance of phenytoin.
Additive hypoglycemic effect with sulfonylurea agents.

Monitor: Temperature, CBC, culture and sensitivity.

VANCOMYCIN (Vancocin, Vancolid)

Pharmacologic Class: Antibacterial agent.

Mechanism of Action: Interferes with bacterial cell-wall synthesis.

Indications: Infections caused by susceptible organisms: *Streptococci, Staphylococci, Clostridium difficile, Corynebacterium, Listeria monocytogenes*.

Routes of Excretion: Almost entirely through renal elimination; half-life 4–8 hr.

Dosage:
IV
  Adult: 2000 mg/d in 2–4 divided doses.
  Pediatric: 44 mg/kg in 2–4 divided doses.
IV—endocarditis prophylaxis
  Adult: 1 g, 0.5–1 hr before procedure.
  Pediatric: 20 mg/kg, 0.5–1 hr before procedure.
Oral—for treatment of enterocolitis due to staphylococci or *Clostridium difficile*
  Adult: 2000 mg/d in 2–4 divided doses.
  Pediatric: 44 mg/kg in 2–4 divided doses.
Reduce dose with renal insufficiency.

Adverse Reactions: Ototoxicity; **flushing** of skin, neck, and shoulders (red-neck syndrome), rash, urticaria, fever, allergic reaction; hypotension; nausea; **nephrotoxicity**; leukopenia; **phlebitis**.

Precautions:
Hypotension, "red-neck syndrome," and urticaria may be minimized by IV administration over 60 minutes.
Use cautiously in patients with renal impairment, previous hearing loss.

Contraindications: Hypersensitivity.

Drug Interactions: Potential increased toxicity with ototoxic and nephrotoxic drugs.

Monitor: Temperature, WBC, culture and sensitivity, vancomycin levels (therapeutic 5–40 mcg/ml).

VERAPAMIL (Calan, Isoptin)

Pharmacologic Class: Calcium channel antagonist, coronary vasodilator.

Mechanism of Action: Coronary vasodilation due to inhibition of calcium entry into vascular and myocardial smooth muscle. Also decreases SA and AV conduction, prolongs refractory periods at AV node.

Indications:
Angina pectoris.
Hypertension.
Arrhythmias.

Route of Excretion: Metabolized by the liver to weakly active metabolites which are usually eliminated; half-life 3.5–12 hr.

Dosage:
Oral: 240–480 mg/d in 3–4 divided doses.
IV
   Adult: 5–10 mg IV over 2 minutes, may repeat 10 mg in 30 min.
   Children (1–15 yr): 0.1–0.3 mg/kg (max 5 mg) over 2 minutes, MR in 30 min.
   Children (<1 yr): 0.1–0.2 mg/kg over 2 min, may repeat in 30 min.

Adverse Reactions: **Dizziness, fatigue, headache; hypotension, edema, bradycardia,** CHF, third-degree AV block, syncope, asystole; nausea, abdominal pain, **constipation;** rash, alopecia.

Precautions:
Hypotension and arrhythmias more likely with IV verapamil. Monitor patient closely.
Use cautiously in patients with CHF, liver or renal disease.

Contraindications: Severe CHF, bradycardia, heart block, sick sinus syndrome, hypersensitivity.

Drug Interactions:
Increased digoxin levels.
Decreased clearance of verapamil by cimetidine, propranolol.
Increased clearance of verapamil by phenytoin, phenobarbital.
Increased risk of CHF with disopyramide and beta blockers.
Additive hypotension with antihypertensives, nitrates, quinidine.

Monitor: Heart rate, blood pressure.

VINBLASTINE (Velban)

Pharmacologic Class: Vinca alkaloid.

Mechanism of Action: Interferes with mitosis and nucleic acid synthesis.

Indications: Antineoplastic used in combination therapy for treatment of lymphomas, mycosis fungoides, Kaposi's sarcoma, and carcinoma of breast and testis.

Route of Excretion: Metabolized by the liver to an active metabolite. Biliary and renal excretion. Half-life 19–24 hr.

Dosage:
IV
  Adults: 3.7 mg/m^2, increase by 1.8 mg/m^2 weekly to maximum dose 18.5 mg/m^2.
  Children: 2.5 mg/m^2, increase by 1.25 mg/m^2 weekly to maximum dose 12.5 mg/m^2.

Adverse Reactions: Peripheral neuropathy, paresthesias, headache, diminished reflexes, depression, seizures; **nausea, vomiting,** abdominal pain, diarrhea, anorexia, constipation, stomatitis; hyperuricemia; **leukopenia,** thrombocytopenia, anemia; alopecia, vesiculation; phlebitis, cellulitis.

Precautions: Use cautiously in patients with decreased bone marrow reserve, women of childbearing potential.

Contraindications: Leukopenia, infections, pregnancy, lactation.

Drug Interactions:
Additive bone marrow depression with other antineoplastics or radiation therapy.
Increased risk of bronchospasm in patients treated with mitomycin.
Raynaud's phenomenon in patient with testicular cancer, treated with bleomycin and vinblastine.

Monitor: CBC.

VINCRISTINE (Oncovin)

Pharmacologic Class: Vinca alkaloid.

Mechanism of Action: Interferes with mitosis and nucleic acid synthesis.

Indications:
Antineoplastic agent used in combination therapy for treatment of acute leukemias, lymphomas, sarcomas, neuroblastoma, and Wilm's tumor.
Idiopathic thrombocytopenic purpura.

Route of Excretion: Primarily hepatically metabolized and eliminated by biliary excretion; $t^{1/2}$ 2.5–5.1 hr.

Dosage:
IV
  Adult: 1.4 mg/m^2.
  Pediatric: 2.0 mg/m^2 weekly.
Reduced dose with liver dysfunction.

Adverse Reactions: Ataxia, **peripheral neuropathy,** paresthesia, headache, diminished reflexes, seizures; diarrhea, abdominal pain, stomatitis, constipation, ileus; atonic bladder, SIADH, hyponatremia, uric acid nephropathy, hyperuricemia; **alopecia;** optic atrophy, diplopia; **phlebitis.**

Precautions:
Use cautiously in patients with infection or leukopenia, hepatic impairment, neuromuscular disease or receiving other neurotoxic drugs, and women of childbearing potential.
Does not cross blood-brain barrier for patients with CNS leukemia.
Do not administer vincristine intrathecally. Additional agents may be required.

Contraindications: Hypersensitivity, patients with Charcot-Marie-Tooth syndrome.

Drug Interactions: Increased risk of bronchospasm in patients treated with mitomycin.

Monitor: Neurologic function.

WARFARIN (Coumadin, Panwarfin, Athrombin K)

Pharmacologic Class: Oral anticoagulant.

Mechanism of Action: Interferes with synthesis of vitamin-K-dependent clotting factors (II, VII, IX, X).

Indications:
Prevention and treatment of venous thrombosis and pulmonary embolism.
Treatment of embolization associated with atrial fibrillation.
Adjunctive therapy for coronary occlusion.
Prevention of thrombus formation and embolization after prosthetic valve placement.

Pharmacodynamics: Onset 8–12 hr; peak 1.5–3 days; duration 2–5 days.

Route of Excretion: Metabolized by the liver; half-life 1.5–3 days.

Dosage: Adjust to maintain PT 1.5–2.5 times control; 10–15 mg/d for 3–4 days, then usually 2.5–10 mg/d.

Adverse Reactions: Hemorrhage; GI, renal, or uterine **bleeding**; nausea, vomiting, anorexia, abdominal cramps, diarrhea, hepatitis; alopecia, rash, urticaria, purple toes; priapism; fever; blood dyscrasias; teratogenesis (fetal warfarin syndrome).

Precautions: Use cautiously in elderly, alcoholics, patients with renal failure, hepatic disease, diabetes, active TB, history of ulcer disease, psychosis, women during menstruation and postpartum period.

Contraindications: Hemophilia, thrombocytopenia; active bleeding, open wounds; active peptic ulcer disease; uncontrolled hypertension; open wound; pregnancy, lactation; threatened abortion; cerebral aneurysm; recent brain, spinal cord, or eye surgery.

Drug Interactions:
Enhanced hypoprothrombinemic effects by
  (1) Inhibition of metabolism by allopurinol, chloramphenicol, cimetidine, disulfiram, ethanol, erythromycin, metronidazole, miconazole, oxyphenbutazone, phenylbutazone, sulfinpyrazone, sulfonamides.
  (2) Displaced anticoagulant from protein binding: chloral hydrate, diflunisal, diazoxide, ethacrynic acid, mefenamic acid, salicylates, sulfonamides, sulfonylureas.
  (3) Decreasing vitamin K production: oral antibiotics, aminoglycosides.
  (4) Miscellaneous mechanisms: anabolic steroids, clofibrate, danazol, dextrothyroxine, gemfibrozil, glucagon, influenza vaccine, ketoconazole, sulindac, thyroid preparations, vitamin E.

Increased bleeding tendencies by
- (1) Antiplatelet agents: salicylates, sulfinpyrazone, dipyridamole, NSAIDs.
- (2) Inhibition of procoagulant factors: quinidine, quinine.
- (3) Increased risk of GI bleeding: salicylates, corticosteroids, potassium chloride, NSAIDs.

Decreased anticoagulant effect by
- (1) Enhanced metabolism by barbiturates, carbamazepine, ethchlorvynol, glutethimide, griseofulvin, nafcillin, phenytoin, rifampin.
- (2) Decreased anticoagulant absorption: aluminum hydroxide, cholestyramine, colestipol.
- (3) Increased procoagulant effect by oral contraceptives, corticosteroids, vitamin K.

Monitor: PT (1.5–2.5 times control), signs of blood loss/bleeding; hemoglobin.

GENERIC/TRADE/CLASSIFICATION INDEX

Generic drugs are lowercase; trade name drugs are capitalized; classifications are *italic*.

acebutolol, 31
ACE inhibitors, 35
acetaminophen, 21
acetylsalicylic acid, 29
Achromycin, 126
Adalat, 91
α_1- *and* α_2-*adrenoceptor antagonists*, 44, 85
Adriamycin, 57
Adrucil, 60
Advil, 69
Aldactone, 120
Aldomet, 85
alkylating agents, 45
allopurinol, 22
Alternagel, 23
Alucaps, 23
aluminum carbonate, 23
aluminum hydroxide, 23
Alupent, 81
Alutabs, 23
Amcill, 28
Amethopterin, 83
amikacin, 63
amiloride, 24
aminoglycosides, 63
Aminophylline, 127
amitriptyline, 25
amoxicillin, 28
Amphogel, 23
amphotericin B, 27
ampicillin, 28
Anacin-3, 21
Ancef, 37
antacids, 23, 34, 87, 118
antianemics, 59
antiarrhythmics, 50, 78, 103, 110, 112, 114, 132
antibiotics, 28, 32, 37–39, 43, 58, 63, 70, 90, 92, 96, 99, 122, 123, 126, 130, 131
anticoagulants, 65, 135
anticonvulsants, 36, 49, 101, 103
antidepressants, 25, 128
antidiarrheals, 54
antiemetics, 86, 111
antifungals, 27, 97
antigout agents, 22, 109
antihistamines, 53

antihypertensive agents, 31, 35, 44, 61, 66, 67, 75, 85, 88, 95, 106, 112
anti-inflammatory drugs, 21, 29, 69, 71
antimanic agents, 79
antimetabolites, 60, 83
antineoplastics, 45, 57, 60, 83, 124, 133, 134
antiparkinson agents, 53, 76
antiplatelet agents, 29
antipsychotics, 40, 64, 111
antipyretics, 21, 29
antituberculars, 73, 117
antitumor antibiotics, 57
antitussives, 53
antiulcer agents, 23, 42, 116, 121
Apogen, 63
Apresoline, 66
ASA, 29
aspirin, 29
atenolol, 31
Athrombin K, 135
Azaline, 122
Azlin, 32
azlocillin, 32
Azulfidine, 122
bacampicillin, 28
Bactrim, 130
Basaljel, 23
Bayer, 29
Benadryl, 53
bendroflumethiazide, 67
Benemid, 109
Benylin, 53
benzathine, 99
benzthiazide, 67
beta-adrenoceptor antagonists, 31, 75, 112
Bicillin LA, 99
bisacodyl, 33
Brethaire, 125
Brethine, 125
Bricanyl, 125
Bristagen, 63
bronchodilators, 81, 125, 127
Bronkodyl Elixophyllin, 127
Calan, 132
Calciparine, 65
calcium carbonate, 34

137

calcium channel antagonists, 51, 91, 132
Capoten, 35
captopril, 35
Carafate, 121
carbamazepine, 36
carbapenems, 70
carbenicillin, 32
cardiac glycosides, 50
Cardioquin, 114
Cardizem, 52
Catapres, 44
cefaclor, 37, 38
cefadroxil, 37
cefamandole, 38
cefazolin, 37
cefonicid, 38
cefoperazone, 39
ceforanide, 38, 39
cefotaxime, 39
cefotetan, 39
cefoxitin, 38
ceftazidime, 39
ceftizoxime, 39
ceftriaxone, 39
cefuroxime, 38
cephalexin, 37
cephalosporins, 37-39
cephalothin, 37
cephapirin, 37
cephradine, 37
chlorothiazide, 67
chlorpromazine, 40
chlortetracycline, 126
chlorthalidone, 67
Chooz, 34
Cibalith S, 79
cimetidine, 42
Cin Quin, 114
Cleocin, 43
clindamycin, 43
clonidine, 44
cloxacillin, 90
Colace, 55
Compazine, 111
coronary vasodilators, 52, 74, 91, 93, 132
Co-Trimoxazole, 130
Coumadin, 135
Crysticillin, 99
Cyclopar, 126
cyclophosphamide, 45
cyclosporine, 46
cyclothiazide, 67
Cytoxan, 45
Datril, 21
Decadron, 47
Deltasone, 107
demeclocycline, 126
Demerol, 80
desipramine, 25
Desyrel, 128
dexamethasone, 47
diazepam, 49
dicloxacillin, 90
digoxin, 50
Dilantin, 103

diltiazem, 52
diphenhydramine, 53
diphenoxylate with atropine, 54
diuretics, 24, 61, 67, 120, 129
docusate, 55
docusate calcium, 55
docusate sodium, 55
Dolophine, 82
dopamine, 56
doxepin, 25
Doxinate, 55
doxorubicin, 57
doxycycline, 126
Dulcolax, 33
Durquin, 114
Dyazide, 129
Dyrenium, 129
Ecotrin, 29
EES, 58
Elavil, 25
electrolytes/electrolyte modifiers, 23, 34, 118, 119
E-Mycin, 58
E-MycinE, 58
enalapril, 35
Endep, 25
Eryc, 58
Erypar, 58
EryPed, 58
Ery-Tab, 58
erythromycin, 58
erythromycin base, 58
erythromycin estolate, 58
erythromycin ethylsuccinate, 58
erythromycin stearate, 58
Esidrix, 67
Eskalith, 79
Ethril, 58
fenoprofen, 69
Feosol, 59
Fergon, 59
Fer-In-Sol, 59
ferrous gluconate, 59
ferrous salts, 59
ferrous sulfate, 59
fluorouracil, 60
Folex, 83
5-FU, 60
Fungizone, 27
Furadantin, 92
furosemide, 61
Gantrisin, 123
Garamycin, 63
Gelusil, 23
gentamicin, 63
glucorticoids, 47, 107
Gulfusin, 123
Haldol, 64
haloperidol, 64
HCTZ, 67
heparin, 65
Hexadrol, 47
hormonal agents, 124
hormones, 72, 77
H_2-receptor antagonists, 42, 116
hydralazine, 66
hydrochlorothiazide, 67

HydroDiuril, 67
ibuprofen, 69
Ilosone, 58
imipenem/dilastatin, 70
imipramine, 25
immunosuppressants, 45, 46, 83
indapamide, 67
Inderal, 112
Indocin, 71
indomethacin, 71
INH, 73
inotropic agents, 50, 56
insulin, 72
Intropin, 56
ISDN, 74
isoniazid, 73
Isoptin, 132
Isordil, 74
isosorbide dinitrate, 74
Kaon Cl, 105
Kayexalate, 119
Kefzol, 37
ketoprofen, 69
K-Lor, 105
Klorvess, 105
Klotrix, 105
K Tab, 105
labetolol, 75
Laniazid, 73
Lanoxin, 50
Lasix, 61
laxatives, 33, 55, 87
Ledercillin K, 99
levodopa/carbidopa, 76
Levothroid, 77
levothyroxine, 77
lidocaine, 78
lincomycin, 43
Liquaemin, 65
lisinopril, 35
Lithane, 79
lithium, 79
lithium carbonate, 79
lithium citrate, 79
Lithobid, 79
Lithonate, 79
Lomotil, 54
Loniten, 88
loop diuretics, 61
Luminal, 101
Maalox, 23
Macrodantin, 92
magaldrate, 23
Magnesium Hydroxide, 87
magnesium hydroxide and aluminum hydroxide, 23
Maxzide, 129
Mefoxin, 38
meperidine, 80
mephobarbital, 101
Metaprel, 81
metaproterenol, 81
methacycline, 126
methadone, 82
metharbital, 101
methicillin, 90
methotrexate, 83

methyclothiazide, 67
α-methyldopa, 85
Meticorten, 107
metoclopramide, 86
metolazone, 67
metoprolol, 31
Mexate, 83
mezlocillin, 32
Micro K, 105
Midamor, 21
milk of magnesia, 87
Minipress, 106
minocycline, 126
minoxidil, 88
Mol Iron, 59
MOM, 87
morphine sulfate, 89
Motrin, 69
moxalactam, 39
MSIR, 89
MTX, 83
Mycostatin, 97
Mylanta, 23
nafcillin, 90
naproxen, 69
Neosar, 45
netilmicin, 63
nifedipine, 91
Nilstat, 97
Nipride, 95
Nitrobid, 93
Nitrodisc, 93
Nitro Dur, 93
Nitrofuran, 92
nitrofurantoin, 92
nitroglycerin, 93
nitroprusside, 95
Nitropress, 95
Nitrospan, 93
Nitrostat, 93
Nolvadex, 124
nonnarcotic analgesics, 21, 29, 69, 71
nonsteroidal anti-inflammatory drugs, 29, 69, 71
norfloxacin, 96
Normodyne, 75
Noroxin, 96
nortriptyline, 25
Nuprin, 69
Nydrazid, 73
nystatin, 97
Omnipen, 28
Oncovin, 134
opioid analgesics, 80, 82, 89, 98
oral calcium salts, 34
Orasone, 107
Oretic, 67
oxacillin, 90
oxycodone, 98
oxytetracycline, 126
Panadol, 21
Panmycin, 126
Panwarfin, 135
paracetamol, 21
Pediamycin, 58
Penapar VK, 99

139

penicillin G, 99
penicillins, 28, 32, 90, 99
penicillin V, 99
Pentids, 99
Pen Vee K, 99
Percocet, 98
Percodan, 98
Percodan-Demi, 98
Permapen, 99
Pfizerpen, 99
phenobarbital, 101
phenytoin, 103
Phyllin, 127
piperacillin, 32
Polycillin, 28
Polycyline, 126
potassium chloride, 105
Potassium-Dialose, 55
potassium-sparing diuretics, 24, 120, 129
prazosin, 106
prednisone, 107
Primaxin, 70
Principen, 28
probenecid, 109
procainamide, 110
procaine, 99
Procan SR, 110
Procardia, 91
prochlorperazine, 111
Promapar, 40
Promine, 110
Pronestyl, 110
Pronestyl SR, 110
propranolol, 112
protriptyline, 25
Quibron, 127
Quinaglue, 114
quinethazone, 67
Quinidex, 114
quinidine, 114
quinidine gluconate, 114
quinidine polygalacturonate, 114
quinidine sulfate, 114
Quinora, 114
ranitidine, 116
Reglan, 86
Rifadin, 117
rifampin, 117
Rimactane, 117
Riopan, 23
Robicillin VK, 99
Rocephin, 39
Roxanol, 89
Sandimmune, 46
SAS, 122
sedative/hypnotics, 49, 101
Septra, 130
Sinemet, 76
skeletal muscle relaxants, 49
SK-Soxazole, 123
Slow K, 105
sodium bicarbonate, 118
sodium polystyrene sulfonate, 119

Sorbitrate, 74
spironolactone, 120
SPS, 119
sucralfate, 121
sulfasalzine, 122
sulfisoxazole, 123
sulfonamides, 122, 123
sulindac, 71
Sumycin, 126
Surfak, 55
Synthroid, 77
T_4, 77
Tagamet, 42
tamoxifen, 124
Tegretol, 36
Tempra, 21
Tenormin, 31
terbutaline, 125
tetracycline, 126
tetracyclines, 126
Tetracyn, 126
Theobid, 127
TheoDur, 127
Theolair, 127
theophylline, 127
thiazide diuretics, 67
Thorazine, 40
ticarcillin, 32
Titralac, 34
TMP-SMZ, 130
tobramycin, 63
tolmetin, 71
Trandate, 75
Transderm-Nitro, 93
trazodone, 128
triamterene, 129
trimethoprim-sulfamethoxazole, 130
Tums, 34
Tylenol, 21
Tylox, 98
Unipen, 90
Uticillin VK, 99
Valium, 49
Vancocin, 131
Vancolid, 131
vancomycin, 131
vasodilators, 66, 88, 95, 106
vasopressors, 56
V-Cillin K, 99
Veetids, 99
Velban, 133
verapamil, 132
vinblastine, 133
vinca alkaloids, 133, 134
vincristine, 134
warfarin, 135
WinGel, 23
Wyamycin E, 58
Wyamycin S, 58
Wycillin, 99
Xylocaine, 78
Zantac, 116
Zyloprim, 22

140